MCQs for the Cardiology
Knowledge Based Assessment

MCQs for the Cardiology Knowledge Based Assessment

Daniel Augustine

Specialty Trainee Cardiology, Bristol Heart Institute, UK

Paul Leeson

Professor of Cardiovascular Medicine and Consultant Cardiologist, John Radcliffe Hospital and University of Oxford, UK

Ali Khavandi

Consultant Interventional Cardiologist, written while at Bristol Heart Institute, UK

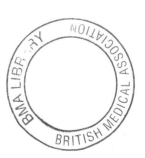

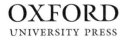

OXFORD
UNIVERSITY PRESS

OXFORD
UNIVERSITY PRESS

Great Clarendon Street, Oxford, OX2 6DP,
United Kingdom

Oxford University Press is a department of the University of Oxford.
It furthers the University's objective of excellence in research, scholarship,
and education by publishing worldwide. Oxford is a registered trade mark of
Oxford University Press in the UK and in certain other countries.

© Oxford University Press 2014

The moral rights of the authors have been asserted

First Edition published in 2014

Impression: 1

Published in the United States of America by Oxford University Press
198 Madison Avenue, New York, NY 10016, United States of America

British Library Cataloguing in Publication Data
Data available

Library of Congress Control Number: 2013938189

ISBN 978–0–19–965551–9

Printed in Great Britain by
Clays Ltd, St Ives Plc

CONTENTS

CONTRIBUTORS

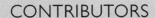

Nauman Ahmed   Cardiology Specialty Trainee, Bristol Heart Institute, UK

Aruna Arujuna   Clinical Research Fellow, Guy's and St Thomas' Hospital NHS Foundation Trust, London, UK

Daniel Augustine   Specialty Trainee Cardiology, Bristol Heart Institute, UK

Richard Bond   BHF Fellow, Bristol University, UK

Dan Bromage   Cardiology Specialty Trainee, Barts Health NHS Trust, UK

William M. Bradlow   Consultant Cardiologist, Queen Elizabeth Hospital, Birmingham, UK

Alan J. Bryan   Cardiac Surgeon, Bristol Heart Institute, Bristol Royal Infirmary, Bristol, UK

Amy Burchell   Cardiology Specialty Trainee, Gloucester Royal Hospital, UK

Stephanie Curtis   Consultant Cardiologist, Adult Congenital Heart Disease, Bristol Heart Institute, UK

Edward J. Davies   Specialist Registrar in Cardiology, Royal Devon and Exeter Foundation Trust, UK

Patrick J. Doherty   Department of Health Sciences, University of York, UK

Timothy A. Fairbairn   Cardiovascular Research Fellow and Cardiology Registrar, University of Leeds, UK

Paul Foley   Consultant Cardiology, Wiltshire Cardiac Centre and Oxford Heart Centre, UK

Oliver E. Gosling   Cardiology MD Fellow, Royal Devon and Exeter NHS Foundation Trust, UK

Rob Hastings   BHF Clinical Research Fellow, Department of Cardiovascular Medicine, University of Oxford, UK

Andy Hogarth   Specialist Registrar, Cardiology, The Yorkshire Heart Centre, Leeds General Infirmary, UK

Yasmin Ismail   Specialist Registrar in Cardiology, Bristol Heart Institute, UK

Paramit Jeetley   Consultant Cardiologist, Bristol Heart Institute, UK

Ali Khavandi   Consultant Interventional Cardiologist, written while at Bristol Heart Institute, UK

Kaivan Khavandi   BHF Academic Clinical Fellow, Guy's and St Thomas' Hospital NHS Foundation Trust, London, UK

Raveen Kandan   Cardiology Speciality Trainee, Royal United Hospital, Bath, UK

Paul Leeson   Professor of Cardiovascular Medicine and Consultant Cardiologist, John Radcliffe Hospital and University of Oxford, UK

Margaret Loudon   Specialist Registrar in Cardiology, Oxford Heart Centre, UK

Nathan Manghat   Consultant Cardiovascular and Interventional Radiologist, Clinical Lead in Cardiac CT, Bristol Heart Institute, Dept of Radiology Bristol Royal Infirmary, UK

Helen Mathias   Consultant Cardiac Radiologist, Queen Elizabeth Hospital Birmingham, UK

Rani Robson   Cardiology Specialist Registrar, Cheltenham General Hospital, UK

James Rosengarten   Specialist Registrar in Cardiology, Southampton General Hospital, UK

Nik Sabharwal   Consultant Cardiologist, Oxford Heart Centre, UK

Anoop K. Shetty   Clinical Research Fellow, Guy's and St Thomas' Hospital NHS Foundation Trust, London, UK

Graham Stuart   Consultant Cardiologist (Paediatric and Adult Congenital Heart Disease), Bristol Heart Institute and Bristol Royal Hospital for Children, Bristol, UK

Ian P. Temple   Cardiology and Electrophysiology Specialist Registrar, BHF Clinical Fellow, The University of Manchester, UK

David Wilson   Cardiology Specialty Trainee, Bristol Heart Institute, Bristol, UK

ABBREVIATIONS

AASK	African American Study of Kidney Disease
ABPM	ambulatory blood pressure monitor
ACE	angiotensin-converting enzyme
ACS	acute coronary syndrome
ADP	adenosine diphosphate
AF	atrial fibrillation
AHA	American Heart Association
AR	aortic regurgitation
ARB	angiotensin-receptor blocker
ARVC	arrhythmogenic right ventricular cardiomyopathy
AS	aortic stenosis
ASD	atrial septal defect
ATP	antitachycardia pacing
AV	atrioventricular
AVNT/AVNRT	atrioventricular re-entrant nodal tachycardia
AVR	aortic valve replacement
AVRT	atrioventricular reciprocating tachycardia
AVSD	atrioventricular septal defect
bd	twice daily (bis in die)
BMI	body mass index
BMS	bare metal stent
BNP	brain natriuretic peptide
BP	blood pressure
bpm	beats per minute
BSA	body surface area
BSE	British Society of Echocardiography
CABG	coronary artery bypass surgery
CACS	coronary artery calcium scoring
ccTGA	congenitally corrected transposition of the great arteries
CCU	cardiac care unit; coronary care unit
CHD	coronary heart disease
CK	creatine kinase
cm	centimetres
CMR	cardiovascular magnetic resonance
CO	cardiac output
COPD	chronic obstructive pulmonary disease

CR	cardiac rehabilitation
CRP	C-reactive protein
CRT	cardiac resynchronization therapy
CRT-D	CRT defibrillator
CRT-P	CRT pacemaker
CT	computed tomography
CTEPH	chronic thromboembolic pulmonary hypertension
CTG	cardiotocography
CVD	cardiovascular disease
CW	continuous wave
Cx	circumflex
CXR	chest X-ray
DAPT	dual-antiplatelet therapy
DBP	diastolic blood pressure
DC	direct current
DES	drug-eluting stent
dL	decilitres
DSE	dobutamine stress echocardiography
ECG	electrocardiogram
ED	emergency department
EF	ejection fraction
eGFR	estimated glomerular filtration rate
EMI	electromagnetic interference
EP	electrophysiology
ERO	effective regurgitant orifice (area)
ESC	European Society of Cardiology
ESR	erythrocyte sedimentation ratio
ETT	exercise treadmill test
FDA	US Food and Drugs Administration
FFR	fractional flow reserve
FH	familial hypercholesterolaemia
g	grams
GCS	Glasgow Coma Score
GI	gastrointestinal
GP	general practitioner; glycoprotein
GTN	glyceryl trinitrate
GUCH	grown-up congenital heart disease
HADS	Hospital Anxiety and Depression Scale
Hb	haemoglobin
HDL	high-density lipid
H-ISDN	hydralazine and isosorbide dinitrate
HIT	heparin-induced thrombocytopenia
IAS	inter-atrial septum
ICD	implantable cardioverter–defibrillator
IE	infectious endocarditis

IHD	ischaemic heart disease
INR	international normalized ratio
IV	intravenous
IVUS	intravascular ultrasound
JBS	Joint British Societies
JVP	jugular venous pressure
K	potassium
kg	kilograms
L	litres
LA	left atrium
LAD	left anterior descending artery
LAO	left anterior oblique
LBBB	left bundle branch block
LCx	left circumflex artery
LDL	low-density lipid
LDL-C	low-density lipid cholesterol
LGE	late gadolinium enhancement
LIMA	left internal mammary artery
LMS	left main stem
LMWH	low molecular weight heparin
LV	left ventricle/ventricular
LVAD	left ventricular assist device
LVEDD	left ventricular end-diastolic diameter
LVEF	left ventricular ejection fraction
LVH	left ventricular hypertrophy
LVOT	left ventricular outflow tract
LVSD	left ventricular systolic dimension
m/s	metres per second
mA s	milli-ampere seconds
MET	metabolic equivalent of task
mg	milligrams
MI	myocardial infarction
mL	millilitres
μmol	micromoles
mPAP	mean pulmonary artery pressure
MPS	myocardial perfusion scintigraphy
mPWP	mean pulmonary wedge pressure
MR	mitral regurgitation
MRA	magnetic resonance angiography
MRI	magnetic resonance image/imaging
MS	mitral stenosis
ms	milliseconds
MV	mitral valve
MVA	mitral wave area

MVo$_2$	myocardial oxygen consumption
Na	sodium
ng	nanograms
NICE	National Institute for Health and Care Excellence
NO	nitric oxide
nocte	at night
NSF CHD	National Service Framework for Coronary Heart Disease
NSTE-ACS	non-ST elevation acute coronary syndrome
NSTEMI	non-ST segment elevation myocardial infarction
NSVT	non-sustained ventricular tachycardia
NYHA	New York Heart Association
od	once daily
OM	obtuse marginal (coronary artery)
OPAT	outpatient parenteral antibiotic therapy
PAF	paroxysmal atrial fibrillation
PCI	percutaneous coronary intervention
PDA	patent ductus arteriosus
PE	pulmonary embolism
PET	positron emission tomography
PFO	patent foramen ovale
pg	picograms
PH	pulmonary hypertension
PHT	pressure half-time
PISA	proximal isovelocity surface area
PPAR	peroxisome proliferator-activated receptor
PPI	proton pump inhibitor
PVI	pulmonary vein isolation
PW	pulsed wave
RAO	right anterior oblique
RAP	right atrial pressure
RBBB	right bundle branch block
RCA	right coronary artery
RIMA	right internal mammary artery
RNV	radionuclide ventriculography
RV	right ventricle/ventricular
RVEF	right ventricular ejection fraction
RVOT	right ventricular outflow tract
RWMA	right wall motion abnormality
SAM	systolic anterior motion
SBP	systolic blood pressure
SCD	sudden cardiac death
SHO	senior house officer
STEMI	ST elevation myocardial infarction
SVT	supraventicular tachycardia
TAPSE	tricuspid annular plane systolic excursion

TAVI	transcatheter aortic valve implantation
TC	total cholesterol
TCPC	total cavopulmonary connection
TOD	target organ damage
TOE	transoesophageal echocardiogram
ToF	tetralogy of Fallot
TR	tricuspid regurgitation
TTE	transthoracic echocardiogram
U&E	urea and electrolytes
UFH	unfractionated heparin
UTI	urinary tract infection
VC	vena contracta
VF	ventricular fibrillation
VSD	ventricular septal defect
VT	ventricular tachycardia
WCC	white cell count

1. **A patient is diagnosed with long QT syndrome and has been commenced on beta-blockers with no symptoms and a QTc of 470 ms. No genetic testing has been performed. She has a 7-year-old daughter and asks about the risks for her child.**

    What is it appropriate to tell her?

    A. The patient should be considered for genetic testing
    B. The patient's daughter should be considered for genetic testing
    C. An ICD is likely to be the safest option
    D. If her daughter has a normal ECG she can be reassured that she does not have long QT syndrome
    E. No further investigation is necessary

2. **A 61-year-old with a history of a myocardial infarction 2 years ago with a known ejection fraction of 25% presents to A&E with a 2 hour history of mild palpitations. He is otherwise fit and well. His ECG monitoring shows a regular broad complex tachycardia at a rate of 170 bpm which self-terminated before a 12-lead ECG was performed. His U&Es are normal. The patient's blood pressure was 130/90 mmHg during the tachycardia and he was not unduly distressed. He is transferred to CCU where a 12-lead ECG shows LBBB with a QRS duration of 100 ms.**

    A. He needs an ICD
    B. He needs an urgent revascularization
    C. He needs an EP study
    D. He tolerated his tachycardia well; therefore it is likely to be an SVT with aberrancy
    E. He should be commenced on flecainide

3. **A patient with previous myocardial infarction, an ejection fraction of 25%, and a QRS duration of 140 ms, but no history of cardiac arrest, is seen in clinic and an ICD is recommended. She is concerned about driving.**

    What is it appropriate to tell her?

    A. She will need to stop driving for 6 months
    B. She will need to stop driving for 1 month
    C. If she has an appropriate shock she will need to stop driving for 6 months
    D. A and C
    E. B and C

4. **Which one of the following features is least suggestive that a broad complex tachycardia is ventricular in origin (VT)?**
    A. P waves seen 'walking through the tachycardia'
    B. The QRS duration shortens as the patient goes from sinus rhythm to tachycardia
    C. Capture beats
    D. A right bundle branch block pattern with a small R wave and a large R' wave (i.e. rsR') in V1
    E. Negative concordance in the chest leads

5. **A 37-year-old man presents to A&E with pneumonia and a temperature of 39°C. He has no chest pain but a routine ECG is performed and is shown in Figure 1.1.**
    A. He should be referred for primary angioplasty
    B. His temperature may have exacerbated his ECG changes
    C. He should be treated with ajmaline
    D. He needs an ICD
    E. Beta-blockers are indicated

6. **Which one of the following would not be considered a high-risk marker for sudden cardiac death in hypertrophic cardiomyopathy?**
    A. Family history of sudden cardiac death
    B. Non-sustained VT on cardiac monitoring
    C. LV septal thickness of 2.3cm
    D. Drop in blood pressure on ETT
    E. Syncope

7. **A 26-year-old patient presents to A&E with the rhythm strip shown in Figure 1.2. He is complaining of palpitations and chest pain. His blood pressure is 80/60 mmHg.**

    What should the initial management be?
    A. IV adenosine
    B. IV amiodarone
    C. IV beta-blocker
    D. IV calcium-channel blocker
    E. Urgent cardioversion

8. **The ECG shown in Figure 1.2 is diagnostic of which one of the following rhythms?**
    A. AF with aberrancy
    B. AF with pre-excitation
    C. VT
    D. AVNT—orthodromic
    E. AVNT—antidromic

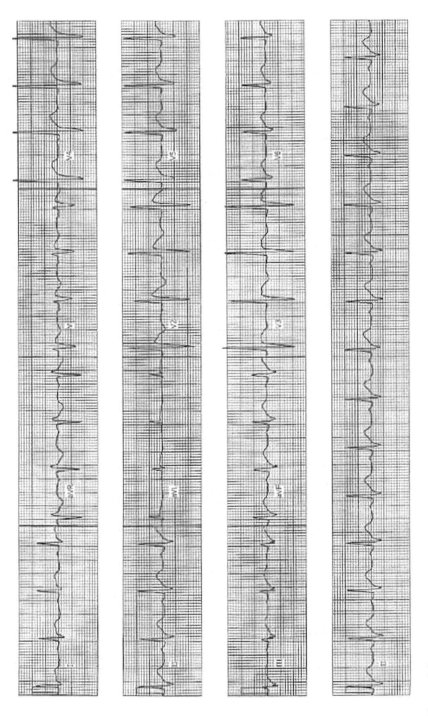

Figure 1.1

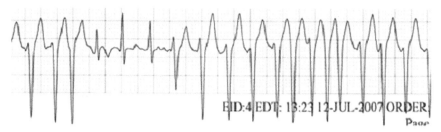

Figure 1.2

9. **Which one of these drugs does not prolong the QT interval?**
   A. Amiodarone
   B. Erythromycin
   C. Carbemazpine
   D. Clozapine
   E. Methadone

10. **What does the the box plot in Figure 1.3 show?**
   A. An inappropriate shock for AF
   B. Inappropriate ATP for AF
   C. Appropriate shock for VT
   D. Appropriate ATP for VT
   E. Appropriate shock for VF

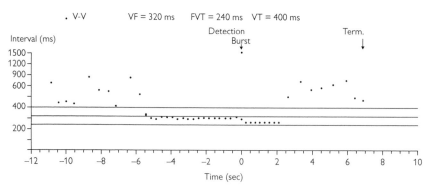

Figure 1.3

11. **With regard to ARVC:**
   A. The diagnosis can be confirmed on the basis of MRI findings alone
   B. All patients with a confirmed diagnosis will need an ICD
   C. It is normally autosomal dominant
   D. Genetic tests are positive in most cases
   E. A and C

12. **A 57-year-old patient with a history of dilated cardiomyopathy and an ejection fraction of 20% is admitted to hospital after a presyncopal episode. His ECG on arrival shows monomorphic VT with a rate of 180 bpm and his BP is 70/50 mmHg. He receives urgent cardioversion and his QRS complexes are narrow on return to sinus rhythm. He is normally NYHA class III and is on maximum medication for HF.**

    A. According to NICE criteria he does not qualify for an ICD as his aetiology is not IHD
    B. He should receive a biventricular ICD
    C. He should receive a standard ICD
    D. He should be commenced on oral amiodarone
    E. He should be considered for a VT ablation

13. **An asymptomatic 32-year-old man has the ECG shown in Figure 1.4 performed as part of a routine work medical examination.**

    A. This ECG shows right bundle branch block
    B. He is asymptomatic and can be reassured without further investigation
    C. He should have a 5 day monitor and as long as there are no significant arrhythmias or changes in the QRS complexes he can be reassured and discharged
    D. He should have an echocardiogram and if this is normal he can be reassured and discharged
    E. He should proceed to an EP study

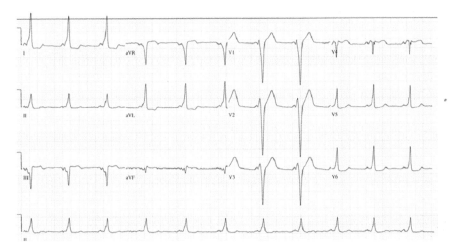

Figure 1.4

14. What is the rhythm shown in Figure 1.5?

A. AF with pre-existing RBBB

B. AVNRT with aberrancy

C. VT—likely to arise from the left ventricle

D. VT—likely to arise from the right ventricle

E. Antidromic AVRT

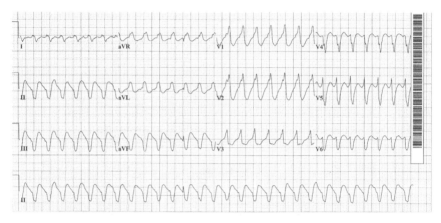

Figure 1.5

15. A patient with a secondary prevention ICD *in situ* experienced a shock from his device. The download is shown in Figure 1.6. It is a single-chamber device and the top trace is from the RV tip to RV ring and the lower trace is from the generator can to the RV shock coil.

A. He has had an appropriate shock for VF

B. He has had VF appropriately terminated with ATP

C. He has had VT appropriately terminated with ATP

D. He has had an inappropriate shock

E. The arrhythmia has self-terminated

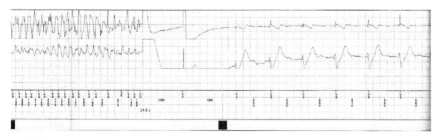

Figure 1.6

16. **A 65-year-old diabetic man with a previous history of myocardial infarction 3 years ago (no intervention required) is found to have atrial fibrillation. His LVEF is 55% and he has no cardiovascular symptoms.**

    What would you advise him with regard to the best thromboprophylaxis?

    A. High-dose aspirin
    B. Aspirin and clopidogrel
    C. Aspirin and warfarin
    D. Aspirin or warfarin
    E. Warfarin

17. **A 25-year-old man presents to the ED with a broad complex tachycardia that is irregularly irregular. The patient is haemodynamically uncompromised. An anaesthetist is not available to assist with immediate DC cardioversion.**

    What is the best initial treatment option?

    A. IV adenosine
    B. IV verapamil
    C. Oral beta-blocker
    D. IV beta-blocker
    E. IV flecainide

18. **A 60-year-old man attends clinic because of hypertension. His BP in clinic is 170/90 mmHg and his echocardiogram shows mild LVH and mild LA dilatation. He is not diabetic and has no other medical history of note.**

    Which one of the following medications is most effective in preventing AF?

    A. ACE inhibitors
    B. Beta-blockers
    C. Calcium-channel antagonists
    D. Diuretics
    E. Alpha-blockers

19. **A 62-year-old woman attends clinic following an ED attendance 6 weeks previously with a one-week history of palpitations. She was diagnosed with AF at the time and commenced on aspirin and a beta-blocker. Her echocardiogram showed no significant abnormalities and her ECG in clinic today confirms atrial fibrillation with a ventricular rate of 70 bpm. She continues to get occasional palpitations and would like to be considered for cardioversion.**

    What do you advise?

    A. She needs to be warfarinized for at least 48 hours pre-cardioversion
    B. Anticoagulation should be continued after successful cardioversion for at least 4 weeks
    C. If a TOE rules out atrial thrombus, no anticoagulation is required post-procedure
    D. Anticoagulation is not required prior to chemical cardioversion
    E. Anticoagulation is not required prior to cardioversion as her CHADS2 score is zero

20. **A 75-year-old diabetic woman with a history of previous MI and an LVEF of 35% has been on amiodarone for paroxysmal AF for several years. On examination she is breathless at rest and has signs of congestive cardiac failure. She has heard about dronedarone and is wondering whether she can have it instead of amiodarone.**

    What do you advise her about dronedarone?

    A. It is more effective than amiodarone in maintaining sinus rhythm
    B. It has no effect on heart (ventricular) rate during AF episodes
    C. It is contraindicated in NYHA class IV heart failure patients
    D. It is suitable for her as she is diabetic and aged over 70
    E. It is associated with more ocular side effects than amiodarone

21. **A 66-year-old woman with a past medical history of hypertension undergoes DC cardioversion for atrial fibrillation. Immediately following the procedure, transient ST elevation is seen. The patient is asymptomatic post-procedure but cardiac enzymes are taken 12 hours later. These show a normal troponin I but a raised CK. The SHO calls you to advise him on the significance of the ECG and blood tests.**

    What do you advise?

    A. The ST elevation and raised CK are probably not abnormal
    B. A rise in troponin I, but not in troponin T, is sometimes seen following AF cardioversion
    C. A rise in troponin T, but not in troponin I, is sometimes seen following AF cardioversion
    D. Both troponin I and T are usually raised post-cardioversion
    E. The raised CK suggests likely myocardial damage

22. **A 40-year-old man presents to A&E with a 12-hour history of sudden-onset palpitations. He has no previous medical history of note and the clinical examination is unremarkable. His troponin is negative. His ECG shows atrial fibrillation with a ventricular rate of 130 bpm, his BP is 110/70 mmHg, and his oxygen saturation is 98%. He has no symptoms associated with his palpitations.**

    What is the best management?

    A. Amiodarone 300 mg IV loading followed by 900 mg over 24 hours
    B. Flecainide 2 mg/kg over 10 minutes followed by oral dose
    C. Digoxin 500 micrograms IV followed by 500 micrograms after 6 hours
    D. Anticoagulate, rate control, and perform DC cardioversion in 6 weeks
    E. Aspirin, atenolol 50 mg od, and review in clinic in 6 weeks

23. **A 72-year-old man with symptomatic persistent atrial fibrillation is admitted for pulmonary vein isolation.**

    Which one of the following statements is most likely to be true?

    A. The risk of stroke is around 5%
    B. The chance of successful ablation of the arrhythmia is around 90% at 1 year
    C. The chance of successful ablation is higher for persistent AF than for paroxysmal AF
    D. The risk of cardiac tamponade is around 5%
    E. The risk of pulmonary vein stenosis is around 5%

24. **A patient is admitted for a DC cardioversion for their persistent atrial fibrillation.**

    Which one of the following statements is true?

    A. Monophasic waveforms are more effective than biphasic waveforms at cardioverting patients
    B. IV flecainide pre-procedure does not increase the chances of electrical cardioversion
    C. The initial success rate is around 50%
    D. Patients do not require anticoagulation prior to cardioversion if their CHADS2 score is ≤1
    E. Increased left atrial size is associated with an increased risk of AF recurrence

25. **A 75-year-old man with a previous history of persistent AF, peptic ulceration, and renal failure (creatinine 220 μmol/L) undergoes elective PCI to his LAD with a bare metal stent (BMS). He was on warfarin for AF prior to his PCI.**

    What is the best combination of drugs immediately following the procedure?

    A. Aspirin, clopidogrel, and warfarin
    B. Aspirin and clopidogrel
    C. Aspirin and warfarin
    D. Clopidogrel and warfarin
    E. Warfarin alone

26. **A 35-year-old man with no past medical history of note and on no regular medication presents to clinic with palpitations. Holter monitoring reveals short-lasting episodes of atrial fibrillation during which he has noted 'a fluttering sensation' in his patient diary.**

    What is the best initial management plan?

    A. Warfarin and atenolol
    B. Amiodarone and aspirin
    C. Refer for pulmonary vein isolation
    D. Flecainide and atenolol
    E. Disopyramide and aspirin

27. **An 80-year-old woman with permanent atrial fibrillation and palpitations attends clinic. She has been in AF for over 10 years and has a left atrial diameter of 5.5 cm. She has high ventricular rates despite being on digoxin 125 micrograms od and atenolol 50 mg od. She has dizzy episodes when she has high ventricular rates and had a pre-syncopal episode 1 month ago. She is keen to consider an AV node ablation.**

    What do you advise?

    A. There is no evidence that this will improve her symptoms
    B. The mortality of the procedure is about the same as for medical treatment of AF
    C. The procedure is contraindicated in patients with heart failure
    D. PVI ablation should be attempted first
    E. A pacemaker is required but will be programmed to minimize right heart pacing

28. **A 50-year-old man with a history of hypertension, diabetes, and persistent atrial fibrillation, for which he is warfarinized, is admitted with an NSTEMI. He undergoes PCI to his proximal LAD with a drug-eluting stent (DES).**

    What is the best combination of drugs following his intervention?

    A. Aspirin, clopidogrel, and warfarin for 1 month; then warfarin alone thereafter
    B. Aspirin, clopidogrel and warfarin for 1 month; then warfarin and clopidogrel for 12 months followed by warfarin alone
    C. Aspirin, clopidogrel, and warfarin for 6 months; then warfarin and clopidogrel for 6 months followed by warfarin alone
    D. Aspirin, clopidogrel and warfarin for 12 months; then warfarin alone
    E. Aspirin and warfarin for 12 months; then clopidogrel alone

29. **An 85-year-old woman is referred to your cardiology clinic because of an incidental finding of atrial fibrillation at a routine check-up. The patient is asymptomatic from a cardiovascular perspective, but a 24-hour tape organized by the GP shows atrial fibrillation throughout with rates varying between 60 and 110 bpm. The patient has a history of hypertension and stable angina. Coronary angiography performed several years ago showed minor atheroma in the LAD, circumflex, and RCA. Echocardiography shows good biventricular systolic function with a left atrial diameter of 5.2 cm. The patient is on aspirin 75 mg od, ramipril 10 mg od, simvastatin 20 mg od, and atenolol 50 mg od.**

    What thromboprophylactic treatment do you recommend?

    A. Warfarinization with a target INR of 2.0–3.0
    B. Warfarinization with a target INR of 1.8–2.5
    C. Continue with aspirin 75 mg od
    D. Aspirin and warfarin with a target INR of 2.0–3.0
    E. Aspirin and warfarin with a target INR of 1.8–2.5

30. **An 18-year-old woman attends the ED with palpitations and dizziness. An ECG shows a broad complex tachycardia with an irregularly irregular rhythm and a ventricular rate of 160 bpm. Her BP is 88/60 mmHg but she has no chest pain or dyspnoea. She had been told several years earlier that she had a 'Wolff–Parkinson–White ECG' and offered 'a procedure' for this but declined. She has had no previous admissions to hospital and is on no regular medication.**

    What is the best treatment?

    A. Adenosine IV
    B. Verapamil IV
    C. Amiodarone IV
    D. Flecainide IV
    E. DC cardioversion

1. A. An increasing number of genes have been identified for the long QT syndrome but approximately 80% of patients have a mutation of one of three genes (LQT1–3). It is always best to perform genetic tests on the subject who has the clearest case of the condition. In this case, this is the patient herself. If a culprit gene can be found, the process of screening family members becomes much simpler.

2. A. This man is very likely to have sustained ventricular tachycardia (VT) given his history of ischaemic heart disease, impaired ejection fraction, and broad complex tachycardia. The fact that he has tolerated it well is not an indication that it is an SVT, although this is possible. Therefore an ICD is indicated by NICE criteria as he has an EF <35%, sustained VT, ischaemic aetiology, and NYHA class III or less. It should be noted that this is a secondary prevention indication despite the fact the patient does not appear to have been compromised by his VT. NICE recommends a VT stimulation study for non-sustained VT (NSVT) and EF <35%, but the patient already meets criteria for an ICD and therefore this would be a redundant investigation. Flecainide is contraindicated in patients with established IHD or structural heart disease.

3. E. The ICD would be a primary prevention device and therefore the patient needs to stop driving for 1 month (compared with 6 months for a secondary prevention device). However, if she has an appropriate shock it is then treated in the same way as a device implanted for secondary prevention and requires 6 months off driving.

4. D. P waves walking through the tachycardia and capture beats are evidence of independent P-wave activity and 'prove' that the rhythm is VT. If the QRS is broad in sinus rhythm, it indicates pre-existing conduction tissue disease which will not shorten if the tachycardia is an SVT. Therefore shortening of the QRS proves that the rhythm is VT, probably originating from the septum to give a relatively narrow QRS. Negative concordance shows that the rhythm is originating from the apex of the heart and is therefore VT. The rsR' pattern is seen in typical RBBB and is suggestive of aberrancy rather than VT, although this is not diagnostic.

5. B. This ECG is highly suggestive of Brugada syndrome with a type 1 pattern, i.e. >2 mm ST elevation in the J point, downsloping ST elevation, and inverted T waves best seen in lead V2. The ECG changes can certainly be brought about by fevers, and therefore B is the correct answer. There is no description of syncope and therefore the patient does not meet the criteria for considering an ICD. Ajmaline is not a treatment for Brugada! It is a test for people with type 2 or type 3 Brugada pattern on ECG to provoke a type 1 pattern, but should not be given to people who already have a type 1 pattern as it may provoke dangerous arrhythmias. There is no well-established medical therapy for Brugada syndrome although trials with quinidine are under way.

6. C. A septal thickness of >3 cm is considered a high-risk marker. All the other factors are high-risk markers.

7. E. See the answer to Question 8 of this chapter for more details.

8. B. The clue to this ECG is the irregular nature of the QRS complexes, although this can be difficult to detect at fast heart rates. AF with aberrancy would also be possible with an irregular rhythm, but this would have a more typical bundle branch block appearance. In a compromised patient with very short RR intervals and broad QRS complexes, pre-excited AF should be presumed. Drugs that block the AV node should be avoided in pre-excited AF as they are ineffective because fast conduction is across the pathway. Drugs which are negatively inotropic, such as calcium-channel blockers and beta-blockers can also lead to worsening haemodynamics and even death and therefore are contraindicated. Intravenous flecainide could be considered as it will slow conduction across the pathway, but this patient's heart is going very fast with symptoms and a low BP, and therefore urgent DC cardioversion should be performed in ED resuscitation.

9. C. The other drugs mentioned are all well known to cause QT prolongation and should be avoided in people with long QT syndrome. Sometimes this is difficult and a risk–benefit decision needs to be made. A full list of drugs known to cause QT prolongation can be found at http://QTdrugs.org.

10. D. This is a single-chamber ICD and therefore there is no information from the atrium. At the beginning of the trace the RR intervals are irregular and relatively long (none are less than 400 ms). This is due to underlying AF. There is then a sudden increase to a regular tachycardia with a cycle length of 300 ms (rate 200 bpm) which is entirely consistent with VT. There are 18 of these beats before the device appropriately detects VT, marked with the word detection appearing at time point 0. The giveaway that ATP is delivered is the word 'Burst' being documented, but it can also be seen that 8 beats occur at a slightly shorter RR interval than the VT before the successful termination of the VT and a return to AF with a slower irregular RR interval. These 8 beats are the ATP being delivered. It is important to scrutinize all the information on the programmer printouts carefully as each manufacturer gives the information in a different format.

11. C. To confirm the diagnosis two major, one major and two minor, or four minor criteria are needed, and therefore a diagnosis cannot be made solely on cardiac MRI. Asymptomatic patients with mild disease do not require an ICD. The condition is usually autosomal dominant, but currently genes are only identified in approximately 30% of cases.

12. C. NICE criteria regarding the need for the aetiology to be IHD only apply in the primary prevention setting, but this case describes the need for secondary prevention. The patient's QRS is narrow; therefore a biventricular pacemaker is not indicated at present and it should be possible to programme the device so that pacing is not needed. The ICD will attempt to treat the monomorphic VT with ATP in this patient, and if this is successful there may well be no need to consider further suppression of VT with either medication or ablation.

13. E. The ECG shows pre-excitation. Even though the patient is asymptomatic there is a risk of SCD due to pre-excited AF. There is no consensus on the best way to risk stratify patients, but if non-invasive testing is preferred a 5-day monitor could be performed. However, its main use is to see whether the pathway is intermittent with a sudden loss of pre-excitation which would place the patient in a lower risk category. In answer C there is no loss of pre-excitation during the 5-day monitor and therefore it would not be reasonable simply to discharge him. EP studies allow risk stratification and then the possibility of ablating a high-risk pathway at the same time.

14. C. This ECG shows a regular broad complex tachycardia. It has several features of VT with an unusual morphology for RBBB, an axis of −90°, and positivity in aVR. The 12th beat is a fusion beat which clinches the diagnosis. The fact that this is 'RBBB-like' suggests that it arises from the left ventricle and then crosses over to the right ventricle in a way that is analogous to conduction in RBBB.

15. A. This is a single-chamber device and it is important not to become confused and think that the top trace is from an atrial lead and that the diagnosis is AF. The rate is very fast and irregular with a chaotic morphology demonstrating VF. ATP would have been unsuccessful, but a further clue that this was a shock comes from the notation 24.9J at the bottom of the strip at the point the shock was delivered. Different manufacturers' interrogation strips can look quite different but close scrutiny of all the information can often give the answer.

16. E. This man has a CHADS2 score of 1 (one point for diabetes) and therefore could be offered warfarin or aspirin thromboprophylaxis according to this risk stratification system. However, if the newer CHA2DS2-VASc system is used, he has a score of 3 (one point for each of DM, age 65–74, and previous MI) and should be offered oral anticoagulation (warfarin or newer agents). A CHA2DS2-VASc score of zero is truly low risk and could be managed with no thromboprophylaxis at all or aspirin (no thromboprophylaxis preferable). A CHA2DS2-VASc score of 1 could be managed with aspirin or oral anticoagulation (the latter is preferable). A score ≥2 should be managed with oral anticoagulation. In summary oral anticoagulation is preferred to aspirin in AF patients with one or more stroke risk factors based on the CHA2DS2-VASc score.

In the absence of recent ACS or coronary artery stenting, there is no good evidence for either warfarin or antiplatelet drugs.

17. E. This man may have an accessory pathway with rapidly conducted AF. Adenosine, digoxin, verapamil, and beta-blockers should all be avoided as they prolong the AV node refractory period and thus may increase conduction down an accessory pathway. This increases the risk of rapidly conducted AF becoming VF. Intravenous class I antiarrhythmic drugs (e.g. procainamide, flecainide, propafenone) can be used as well as amiodarone, but DC cardioversion is the treatment of choice if there is haemodynamic compromise or rapidly conducted AF down an accessory pathway.

18. A. ACE inhibitors and ARBs have antifibrillatory and antifibrotic properties. A meta-analysis has shown that ACE inhibitors and angiotensin-receptor blockers (ARBs) reduce the relative risk of incident AF by 25%. The LIFE study, in particular, showed a 33% reduction in new-onset AF in patients with LVH treated with losartan compared with those treated with atenolol.

19. B. Patients should be anticoagulated with a therapeutic INR (>2) for at least 3 weeks prior to cardioversion. Anticoagulation should be continued for at least 4 weeks post-cardioversion as 'atrial stunning' may occur. Anticoagulation is required prior to both chemical and electrical cardioverison. If a patient has not had oral anticoagulation for at least 3 weeks, it is reasonable to perform DC cardioversion if a TOE rules out left atrial thrombus. However, LMWH should be commenced prior to a TOE-guided cardioversion and continued post-cardioversion until the target INR is reached with oral anticoagulation.

20. C. This woman appears to be in NYHA class IV heart failure and thus dronedarone is contraindicated according to NICE guidelines. Dronedarone is a structural analogue of amiodarone, but does not contain iodine and thus has a lower risk of skin, lung, and eye side effects. The ATHENA study showed a 24% relative risk reduction of the combined endpoint of cardiovascular hospitalization and death compared with placebo (mainly driven by a reduction in cardiovascular hospitalizations, especially for AF). Dronedarone was also found to reduce the ventricular rate response during AF by 10–15 bpm. Dronedarone is contraindicated in NYHA class III–IV heart failure but is recommended by NICE as an option in patients whose AF is not controlled by first-line therapy and who have at least one of the following risk factors: hypertension (requiring at least two different drugs), diabetes, previous TIA/stroke, LA ≥ 50 mm, LVEF ≤ 40%, and ≥70 years old. There is no evidence that dronedarone is more effective than amiodarone at maintaining sinus rhythm.

21. A. Transient ST elevation can be a normal finding post DC cardioversion. A rise in CK is also usually normal but neither troponin T nor troponin I should rise following DC cardioversion of AF.

22. B. The option of anticoagulation, rate control, and DC cardioversion is reasonable if the onset of atrial fibrillation is >48 hours or if unsure of duration. DC cardioversion could be performed immediately as the onset of AF appears to be acute, but there are no signs of haemodynamic compromise and therefore it does not need to be performed as an emergency. Beta-blockers are good for rate control but are less likely to cardiovert a patient to sinus rhythm than other options. Amiodarone is probably the first-choice drug for chemical cardioversion of patients with structural heart disease or heart failure. Digoxin is unlikely to cardiovert a patient to sinus rhythm and may even be profibrillatory. Flecainide is likely to cardiovert this patient faster than any of the other options, and is likely to be safe in a young patient with no evidence of cardiac disease.

23. D. The risk of stroke is around 1%. The risk of pulmonary vein stenosis/occlusion is around 2%. The success rates reported in the literature for persistent AF ablation are 55–80% at 1 year (this includes some patients who have had more than one procedure). The success rate for PAF ablation is higher at 70–90% at 1 year. Cardiac tamponade usually occurs during or very soon after the procedure, and rates as high as 6% have been reported.

24. E. Biphasic waveforms are more effective than monophasic ones, requiring less energy and fewer shocks to cardiovert patients. Pretreatment with IV ibutilide, flecainide, or sotalol has been shown to decrease the energy requirement for DC cardioversion and increase the success rate. The initial success rate for persistent AF cardioversion is around 80%. All patients should be anticoagulated prior to cardioversion for persistent AF regardless of CHADS2 score. Increased left atrial size, duration of AF prior to cardioversion, previous recurrences, reduced LA function, and underlying cardiac disease are all known to increase AF recurrence risk.

25. A. This is a difficult question. This man has a HAS-BLED score of 3 (one point for each of age >65 years, renal failure, and bleeding predisposition), putting him at a high risk of bleeding. However, he also has a significant thromboembolic risk and antiplatelet drugs alone will not protect him from stroke. The ESC guidelines suggest that, ideally, he should have a BMS rather than a drug-eluting stent to reduce the duration of dual antiplatelets, but he will still require a minimum of 28 days triple therapy (2.6–4.6% risk of major bleed at 30 days). However, data now available for newer-generation drug-eluting stents support 3 months DAP only in some cases and so the risk of reintervention/restenosis is also relevant.

26. D. This patient has CHADS2 and CHA2DS2-VASc scores of zero and can reasonably be given aspirin or no thromboprophylactic medication at all (the latter is preferable according to the ESC). Amiodarone has multiple side effects and is best avoided unless structural heart disease or heart failure are present. Beta-blockers, including sotalol, are reasonable first-choice drugs for the maintenance of sinus rhythm, but warfarin is not indicated here. Therefore the best answer is flecainide and atenolol. Flecainide doubles the chance of maintaining sinus rhythm in PAF patients. AV nodal blocking drugs (such as beta-blockers) should be given with flecainide because of the potential for it to convert AF to atrial flutter, which may then be rapidly conducted to the ventricles. Disopyramide is poorly tolerated because of its antimuscarinic side effects. PVI is not a first-line treatment.

27. B. There is evidence that AV node ablation improves exercise tolerance, LVEF, and quality of life. The overall mortality of the procedure at 1 year (6%) is similar to that of antiarrhythmic therapy for AF. AV node ablation with a CRT implant in those with AF and heart failure has been shown to improve LVEF. PVI is not a first-line treatment for AF. The patient will require 100% ventricular pacing!

28. C. This man has CHADS2 and CHA2DS2VASc scores of 2 and is already warfarinized prior to his NSTEMI. He has a HAS-BLED score of 1 (one point for hypertension) and thus is at low risk of bleeding. The ESC guidelines suggest that a patient with a low or intermediate risk of bleeding who undergoes PCI in the context of ACS (with either BMS or DES) should receive 6 months triple therapy of warfarin + aspirin + clopidogrel, with up to 12 months warfarin and clopidogrel (or aspirin) with PPI cover followed by warfarin alone thereafter (also see answer to Question 10).

29. A. This patient has a CHADS2 score of 2 and a CHA2DS2VASc score of 3. Therefore she should be warfarinized. There is no evidence for a lower INR target range for elderly patients, but studies do suggest a twofold increase in the risk of stroke if the INR range is 1.5–2.0. This woman appears to have stable coronary artery disease, and there is no evidence to suggest that adding aspirin to warfarin reduces the risk of stroke or vascular events in this population (although it does increase the bleeding risk). In elderly patients with minimal symptoms it is reasonable not to pursue a rhythm control strategy.

30. E. This is likely to be pre-excited AF and is potentially life-threatening as AF conducted antegradely down an accessory pathway may degenerate into VF. The patient is haemodynamically compromised as she complains of dizziness and is hypotensive. She should undergo DC cardioversion as soon as possible. AV nodal blocking drugs, such as adenosine, digoxin, verapamil, and beta-blockers, should be avoided as they encourage conduction down the accessory pathway.

1. **A 60-year-old hypertensive patient presents to the ED with chest pain. The pain came on very suddenly in the left chest whilst he was lifting a heavy plant pot. The pain is difficult to localize. The intensity has been constant and remains persistent. En route to hospital it has changed location to the left side of the lower thoracic back. He has recently had treatment for thoracic back pain from a chiropractor. He is sweating (looks unwell) and anxious but has no shortness of breath. Blood pressure is 160/90 mmHg, heart rate is 100 bpm and saturations are 99% on room air. The ECG does not show acute ST change. D-dimer is 1700 ng/mL (normal < 500 ng/mL), and troponin is awaited.**

   Based on the information available, what is the most likely diagnosis?

   A. Acute coronary syndrome
   B. Pulmonary embolism
   C. Acute aortic syndrome
   D. Musculoskeletal pain
   E. Pericarditis

2. **You review a 65-year-old male on the post-take ward round who has been referred by his GP with a 2-week history of exertional chest pain. There have been no episodes at rest and he has improved since the GP started him on bisoprolol 2.5 mg od. His resting ECG shows no ischaemia and troponin tests are negative. He has a family history of ischaemic heart disease but no other risk factors.**

   Which investigation would you recommend?

   A. CT coronary angiogram
   B. Invasive coronary angiogram
   C. Exercise treadmill test
   D. Stress echo
   E. Nuclear perfusion scan

3. **A 45-year-old woman presents with ongoing chest pain. Immediate observations reveal BP 140/80 mmHg, heart rate 90 bpm, and saturations 99% on room air.**

    What should you do next?

    A. Administer oxygen
    B. Administer analgesia
    C. Give aspirin 300 mg
    D. Perform a 12-lead ECG
    E. Gain IV access

4. **You review a 55-year-old woman in clinic who has been referred by her GP with recent chest pains. You feel that the nature of the pains is atypical for ischaemia although they are reproduced with exertion. She has no identifiable risk factors for ischaemic heart disease and the resting ECG is normal.**

    What would you recommend?

    A. CT coronary angiogram
    B. Reassure—no further tests required
    C. Invasive coronary angiogram
    D. Exercise treadmill test
    E. Myocardial perfusion scan

5. **Figures 2.1, 2.2, and 2.3 were obtained during angiography of a patient who had redo coronary artery bypass grafting in 1987. He had three grafts and has a recurrence of angina.**

   Interpret Figure 2.1.

   A. Aortic diverticulum
   B. Right coronary graft stump
   C. Left coronary system graft stump
   D. LIMA graft
   E. Aortic pseudoaneurysm

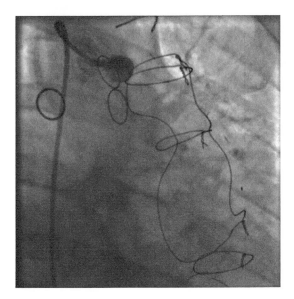

Figure 2.1 RAO angiogram

Answers for Questions 5–7 are given together.

6. Interpret Figure 2.2 for the same patient.

A. Aortic diverticulum

B. Right coronary graft stump

C. Left coronary system graft stump

D. LIMA graft

E. Aortic pseudoaneurysm

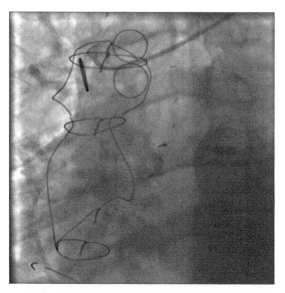

Figure 2.2 LAO angiogram

7. **Interpret Figure 2.3 for the same patient.**

   A. 1 = right subclavian artery, 2 = common carotid artery, 3 = left subclavian artery
   B. 1 = brachiocephalic artery, 2 = right subclavian artery, 3 = left subclavian artery
   C. 1 = right carotid artery, 2 = brachiocephalic artery, 3 = left subclavian artery
   D. 1 = right subclavian artery, 2 = left subclavian artery, 3 = brachiocephalic artery
   E. 1 = brachiocephalic artery, 2 = left carotid artery, 3 = left subclavian artery

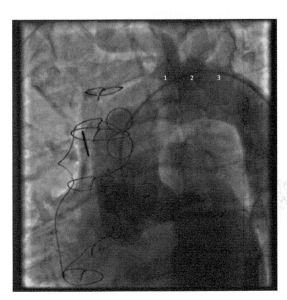

Figure 2.3 Aortogram in LAO

8. **You are referred a 40-year-old lady with left arm pain. She had a single episode after running for a bus with shopping, which subsided after 5 minutes. She has never previously had exertional chest discomfort. Resting ECG is normal and 8 hours high-sensitivity troponin is negative. She has a BMI of 33 and diet-controlled type 2 diabetes mellitus but is not hypertensive.**

   What do you recommend?

   A. Reassure and discharge
   B. Inpatient invasive coronary angiogram
   C. Outpatient stress echo
   D. Discharge-dependent exercise treadmill test
   E. CT coronary angiogram

9. **A 25-year-old male developed sharp central chest pain and palpitations after drinking three cans of energy drink whilst revising for exams. The symptoms were ongoing when he initially attended the ED, and an ECG showed a sinus tachycardia with no ST change. The pain subsided shortly afterwards. He is normally fit and well. His father recently had a myocardial infarction at the age of 62. All observations and examination are normal. Troponin and D-dimer tests were negative.**

What would you recommend?

A. Admit for observations
B. Exercise treadmill test
C. Stress echocardiogram
D. CT coronary angiogram
E. No further investigation

10. **One of your patients has small vessel coronary disease which is not suitable for revascularization. They are still experiencing class 2 angina particularly in the evening despite bisoprolol 10 mg od. Blood pressure is 135/90 mmHg.**

What would you recommend next?

A. Amlodipine
B. Ivabradine
C. Nicorandil
D. Bisoprolol 5 mg bd
E. Ranolazine

11. **One of your patients has discrete angiographically significant lesions in the mid right coronary artery and the mid left anterior descending coronary artery. He is 60 years old and is not diabetic. He has ongoing class 2 anginal symptoms despite optimal dose of a beta-blocker and a long-acting nitrate.**

What do you recommend?

A. CABG will be associated with a greater mortality benefit compared with PCI
B. The risk of stroke will be significantly lower with PCI
C. Add a third oral antianginal and then reconsider revascularization
D. The likelihood of repeat revascularization is higher with PCI
E. Revascularization is recommended for prognostic reasons

12. **A 45-year-old diabetic male patient has returned to clinic following a recent angiogram. He has stable class 2 angina and is currently on aspirin 75 mg od, atorvastatin 40 mg nocte, and bisoprolol 2.5 mg as antianginal treatment. His symptoms have improved since starting the beta-blocker. The angiogram showed severe plaque in the proximal left anterior descending artery and discrete simple lesions in the mid circumflex and right coronary arteries. The echocardiogram has shown moderate LV impairment.**

    What do you recommend?

    A. Titrate the beta-blocker and add a calcium-channel blocker or long-acting nitrate—reassess symptoms

    B. Titrate the beta-blocker and add an ACE inhibitor—reassess symptoms and LV function

    C. CABG for prognostic and symptomatic improvement

    D. PCI guided by ischaemia via a functional imaging test

    E. Multivessel PCI or CABG for symptomatic treatment

13. **Which one of the following is true of atherosclerotic plaque formation?**

    A. It is an acute inflammatory disease of the vascular intima

    B. It is characterized by the accumulation and modification of cholesterol esters on the luminal surface of the endothelium

    C. Macrophages bind and phagocytose oxidized LDL to form foam cells

    D. Typically form away from branch points

    E. Endothelial dysfunction as a result of an insult to the endothelium is characterized by increased nitric oxide release

14. **Atherosclerotic plaque rupture is the most common event leading to clinically relevant ischaemia.**

    Which one of the following statements regarding this process is not true?

    A. Thin-capped fibroatheromas are most prone to cap disruption and thrombus formation

    B. Fracture of the fibrous cap allows platelets, clotting factors, and inflammatory cells to come into contact with the thrombogenic necrotic lipid core, leading to thrombus

    C. Disrupted plaques can be accurately identified by optical coherence tomography

    D. Plaque rupture will always result in some degree of clinical ischaemia (ACS)

    E. Patients presenting with an ACS who have a ruptured plaque identified during angiography can be managed without stenting

15. **Which one of the following statements regarding the new generation of antiplatelet drugs is not true?**

    A. Clopidogrel, prasugrel, and ticagrelor all inhibit the same receptor (P2Y12 ADP receptor)

    B. Clopidogrel and prasugrel are irreversible inhibitors, whereas ticagrelor is reversible

    C. Clopidogrel and prasugrel are both prodrugs which are metabolized to the active form, whereas ticagrelor acts directly

    D. Ticagrelor requires twice daily maintenance, whereas clopidogrel and prasugrel are once daily

    E. All are converted to the active metabolite by the hepatic cytochrome enzyme (CYP3A4) pathway

16. **You are called by the CCU nurses. They are concerned that one of a post primary angioplasty patient's blood results has returned with platelets of 12 × 10⁹/L. Bloods taken at the time of procedure revealed platelets of 179 × 10⁹/L. The patient has no signs of bleeding and all other blood results, including haemoglobin, are stable and consistent. They have been loaded with aspirin 300 mg, prasugrel 60 mg, heparin 8000 units, and abciximab as a weight-adjusted bolus and current infusion for 12 hours. They had not previously received these agents. GP 2b/3a was recommended as the patient had a highly thrombotic right coronary artery occlusion with evidence of microvascular distal embolization and required a long length of drug-eluting stent.**

    What do you advise?

    A. This is likely to be a spurious result; continue with the current treatments but repeat the blood result urgently and watch for bleeding

    B. This degree of platelet inhibition is to be expected with the current regime; reassure but watch for bleeding and repeat the bloods

    C. This is a sign of early heparin-induced thrombocytopenia; stop the abciximab and replace platelets until >50 × 10⁹/L

    D. This may represent an immune-mediated thrombocytopenic reaction to abciximab; stop the infusion and repeat the bloods

    E. The patient is at significant risk of bleeding; stop all antiplatelets until the platelet count is >50 × 10⁹/L

17. **A patient arrives directly in the catheterization laboratory for primary angioplasty. They volunteer a previous serious allergic reaction to heparin called 'HIT' as you are consenting them.**

    What would be your anticoagulation strategy?

    A. A single administration of unfractionated heparin in this situation should be safe

    B. Avoid all anticoagulants as a precaution and complete the procedure with Gb2b/3a cover

    C. Bivalarudin is safe and effective in this situation

    D. A single administration of fondaparinux in this situation should be safe and effective

    E. There is a risk with all anticoagulants in this situation, and so the balance of benefit is shifted to thrombolysis over primary angioplasty

18. You review a patient in clinic who has previously had bypass surgery and a recurrence of angina. They have three grafts (**LIMA** to **LAD**, vein graft to **OM**, and vein graft to **RCA**). You recommend a coronary angiogram. The patient asks you if the procedure will be carried out from the wrist or the leg as they have had vascular procedure to both groins. You can see bilateral inguinal scars, but the procedures were carried out at another hospital.

    What do you advise?

    A. The left wrist would be the preferred route here
    B. The right wrist would be the preferred route here
    C. The left leg would be the preferred route, but you will need to obtain further information regarding the vascular procedures
    D. The right leg would be the preferred route, but you will need to obtain further information regarding the vascular procedures
    E. On further thought an angiogram is not possible and a non-invasive test should be utilized

19. **Which of the following statements is true regarding non-ST elevation acute coronary syndromes (NSTE-ACS) compared with ST elevation myocardial infarctions (STEMI)?**

    A. Initial mortality of NSTE-ACS is higher
    B. Six-month mortality of STEMI is higher
    C. Long-term mortality of NSTE-ACS is higher
    D. STEMI patients are older with more comorbity
    E. STEMI is more frequent

20. On your ward round you review a patient who is 48 hours post anterior **STEMI** treated successfully with primary angioplasty. He has type 2 diabetes and hypertension. He is gradually improving, having initially suffered with heart failure. He still feels 'chesty' and auscultation reveals minimal basal crepitations. Echocardiography has revealed an ejection fraction of 40%. Blood pressure is 110/70 mmHg with heart rate 55 bpm at rest. Ramipril has been titrated to 2.5 mg bd with bisoprolol 2.5mg od. U&Es have remained normal.

    How would you improve his medical treatment?

    A. Add furosemide 40 mg od
    B. Reduce the bisoprolol
    C. Further titrate the ramipril
    D. Add Eplerenone 25 mg od
    E. Add isosorbide mononitrate MR 30 mg od

21. You are asked to review a 32-year-old smoker in the **ED**. He has presented with an hour of ongoing chest pain. The pain is described as left-sided and sharp but not focal. There is no postural change and no change with inspiration. He appears clinically well. The emergency team are concerned because he has anterior **ST** elevation and show you his **ECG** (Figure 2.4).

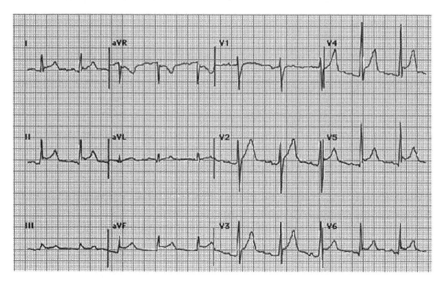

Figure 2.4

What do you recommend?

A. Activation of the primary angioplasty team
B. Await troponin tests and give analgesia
C. Non-steroidal anti-inflammatory analgesia
D. Urgent bedside echo to rule out a regional wall motion abnormality
E. CT pulmonary angiogram

22. **Which of the following should not be used as a procedural antiacoagulant for primary angioplasty?**

A. Unfractionated heparin (± GP 2b/3a)
B. Enoxaparin (± GP 2b/3a)
C. Fondaparinux
D. Bivalarudin
E. Bivalarudin + GP 2b/3a

23. You review a patient in the **CCU** who was admitted earlier with a large anterior myocardial infarction treated with primary angioplasty. He has no bystander disease but the presentation was late. The echocardiogram shows severe **LV** impairment. There is pulmonary oedema which you have been treating with furosemide boluses and continuous positive airway pressure non-invasive ventilation. Blood pressure is now 85/50 mmHg and urine output in the last hour is 10 mL. Oxygen saturations are maintained at 94% with high-flow oxygen. He remains alert.

What treatment should you consider next?

A. Call an anaesthetist to consider ventilation
B. Start a dopamine infusion
C. Give a fluid challenge
D. Start a nitrate infusion
E. Start a furosemide infusion

24. A 45-year-old diabetic man is admitted directly to the catheterization laboratory with chest pain and **ST** elevation. He had elective angioplasty a week previously for stable angina. He received drug-eluting stents and is taking aspirin and clopidogrel. The relevant angiographic image is shown in Figure 2.5.

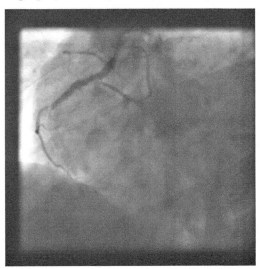

Figure 2.5

What is the diagnosis?

A. Acute stent thrombosis of the right coronary artery
B. Acute stent thrombosis of the left anterior descending artery
C. Acute stent thrombosis of the circumflex artery
D. Acute stent thrombosis of a saphenous vein graft
E. Catheter-induced coronary dissection

25. **You are completing the discharge summary for a patient who has undergone primary angioplasty with a bare metal stent for an anterior myocardial infarction.**

    The pharmacist questions you regarding the duration of antiplatelets. What do you advise?

    A. Dual antiplatelets for 12 months and then aspirin long term

    B. Ticagrelor for 1 month and aspirin long term

    C. Aspirin for 1 month and ticagrelor long term

    D. Ticagrelor alone is adequate long term

    E. Dual antiplatelets long term

1. C.   The question is designed to emphasize the importance of careful history to elicit the pre-test probability of a particular diagnosis. 75% of presentations to the ED with chest pain are of non-ischaemic aetiology. The history is highly suggestive of an aortic syndrome:

- sudden onset (no crescendo as in ACS);
- changing locations (reflecting propagation of dissection);
- hypertensive;
- strongly positive D-dimer (history does not suggest PE; negative D-dimer also has a high negative predictive value for aortic syndromes).

2. B.   The history is very suggestive of stable angina and so the patient has a high likelihood of coronary disease (>90%). Therefore he should go directly to invasive coronary angiography. Exercise treadmill testing is no longer recommended by NICE for stratification of stable angina.

3. D.   An ECG should be performed as soon as possible as prompt diagnosis of ST elevation MI is essential. Nevertheless, the majority of patients presenting with chest pain are of non-ischaemic origin and so the other treatments may not be necessary. If ACS is suspected, aspirin should be given first. Oxygen is not recommended in the chest pain algorithm unless saturations are <94% (aim 94–98% or 88–92% if COPD).

4. A.   This patient has a low probability of coronary disease (10–29%) but may have atypical angina. CT coronary angiogram is the best rule out test.

5. C.

6. B.

7. E.

Questions 5–7 test anatomy common to angiography for graft studies. These images are a particularly good example as graft markers (radio-opaque circles) have been placed and show the graft positions relative to each other in LAO and RAO view.

Right coronary artery grafts are placed above the native RCA on the aorta. The graft is best engaged in the LAO view with the catheter pointing towards the left of the field of view. In this case a stump is revealed at the point of the marker.

Left coronary system grafts (commonly diagonal, obtuse marginal, or intermediate. Vein grafts to the LAD are now uncommon due to the LIMA) are placed sequentially above the native left coronary system. In the RAO view the grafts are engaged with the catheter pointing to the right of the field of view.

The aortogram tests basic aortic arch, head, and neck anatomy. The first branch from the right (1) is the brachiocephalic ('innominate') artery which gives off the right subclavian artery (origin of the RIMA) and right common carotid artery. The middle branch (2) is the left common carotid artery. The third branch (3) is the left subclavian artery which give off the LIMA.

8. C. This woman has an intermediate risk of coronary artery disease (30–60%). She has had a single episode of possible angina but ACS is ruled out. A functional test (stress echo, stress MRI, or nuclear perfusion scan) is the most appropriate form of risk stratification and this can be completed as an outpatient.

9. E. This patient currently has a very low risk of coronary disease (<10%) and so no further ischaemic stratification is necessary. The cause of the symptoms appears to be related to the sinus tachycardia and energy drink. Aggressive primary prevention is, of course, paramount in view of the family history.

10. A. NICE guidelines recommend a beta-blocker **or** a calcium-channel antagonist as first line with the addition of the other class as second line. Third-line agents are long-acting nitrate, iviabradine, nicornadil, or ranolazine.

ESC guidelines marginally select beta-blockers over calcium-channel agonists as first line (evidence is stronger post-MI). Second line in combination with the beta-blocker is a calcium-channel blocker **or** long-acting nitrate. If beta-blockers are contraindicated/not tolerated any class agent can be considered in combination.

Bisoprolol is long acting but atenolol 50 mg bd may be better than 100 mg od because of its shorter half-life. There is clearly blood pressure reserve for amlodipine and the patient may also benefit from improved BP control.

11. D. The benefits of revascularization and the comparison of modalities depend on the patient's background and coronary anatomy. With this anatomy revascularization is for symptoms and not prognosis. Both modalities are equally effective in this respect. Revascularization should be considered for stable angina refractory to two oral antianginals in preference to a third agent. The risk of stroke is similar. Although PCI has the advantage of rapid recovery, the probability of repeat revascularization is statistically higher.

12. C. This question tests an understanding of patterns of stable coronary disease where revascularization is associated with prognostic benefit. The evidence generally favours bypass surgery as the mode of revascularization in these cases. The key features are (1) left main stem disease or (2) multivessel disease with (i) proximal LAD involvement **or** (ii) LV impairment/ large territory of proven ischaemia **or** (iii) in a diabetic patient. The main PCI prognostic indication for stable coronary disease is proven ischaemia with frequent daily symptoms.

13. C. Endothelial injury and dysfunction result from a number of insults. Decreased nitric oxide (NO), which is antiatherogenic, results from endothelial dysfunction. Branch points are vulnerable. Modified cholesterol esters (oxidized LDL) accumulate in the subendothelial space and are phagocytosed by macrophages to form foam cells. Abnormal vascular smooth muscle proliferation at points of atherosclerosis contributes to plaque formation and also determines the stability of the lesions (fibrous cap–thin caps = vulnerability to shear stress).

14. D. Clinically silent plaque rupture with spontaneous healing is well recognized. If a patient presents with an ACS, and a ruptured culprit plaque is identified without luminal stenosis (i.e. ongoing ischaemia), it is reasonable to continue medical therapy without stenting as long as the event has stabilized.

15. E. Clopidogrel and prasugrel are both pro-drugs, irreversible inhibitors, and once-daily regimes. The maintenance dose of prasugrel is halved for weight <60 kg or age >75 years. Clopidogrel is converted to its active metabolite by the cytochrome enzyme pathway; this accounts for the variability of action in some patients (hyporesponders) which can lead to stent thrombosis. Prasugrel is converted to its active form faster and more consistently. Ticagrelor is reversible and direct acting and therefore is again faster acting and more predictable than copidogrel. All inhibit the P2Y12 ADP platelet receptor.

16. D. Inadequate platelet inhibition or platelet replacement will increase the chances of early stent thrombosis and should be avoided. This clinical scenario suggests an early immune-mediated response to abciximab with thrombocytopenia. The platelet count should gradually recover on stopping the agent, but the platelets should not be replaced unless there were signs of significant bleeding.

Heparin-induced thrombocytopenia usually occurs after a few days with repeated exposure.

Pseudo-thrombocytopenia (clumping) is possible and would be obvious on a blood film, but this should be excluded rather than assumed.

17. C. Bivalarudin is a direct thrombin inhibitor and a safe alternative in a patient with previous heparin-induced thrombocytopenia (HIT). The Horizons-AMI trial suggested a significant reduction in all-cause mortality and major bleeding compared with the combination of UFH and GP2b/3a in primary angioplasty patients.

Fondaparinux is a synthetic inhibitor of factor Xa and has been shown not to be inferior to LMWH in ACS, with halved major bleeding (OASIS-5 trial).

18. A. Although, based on the vascular procedure, it is often possible to access the femoral arteries, this is obviously best avoided as there is a greater risk of complications. The left radial will give direct access to the LIMA (comes off the left subclavian artery) and would be the route of choice. The right radial will not allow simple or safe access to the left subclavian artery. If the left radial has been harvested as a graft, then the femoral arteries may have to be considered.

19. C. NSTE-ACS is more frequent with older patients and more comorbidity. Mortality of NSTE-ACS is initially lower, but equal at 6 months and higher in the long term.

20. D. Aldosterone antagonists are indicated if EF ≤ 40% (EPHESUS trial) or if there is heart failure or diabetes, provided that there is no renal failure or hyperkalaemia. The diuretic action should help with the mild residual congestion. Blood pressure will appear to limit further titration of the ACE inhibitor at this stage.

21. D. The diagnosis is uncertain in an acute patient. Pericarditis is more likely, but the anterior ECG changes are most prominent. In the context of ongoing chest pain acute, ischaemia must be urgently ruled out. A bedside echo is the best initial test to exclude a regional wall motion abnormality.

22. C. Use of fondaparinux in the context of primary PCI was associated with potential harm in the OASIS-6 trial and therefore it is not recommended. Bivalarudin is probably the preferred choice currently in primary PCI, but all other options are reasonable. Intravenous enoxaparin is required initially in the context of primary angioplasty.

23. B. This patient has moderate heart failure with pulmonary oedema and significant hypotension. The suggestion is that he may be developing cardiogenic shock. There is evidence of poor organ perfusion, reflected by the urine output, but his ventilation remains reasonable. Inotropic support is the next step. In a patient with BP < 90 mmHg dopamine (inotropic/vasopressor) should be considered. In patients with 'adequate' blood pressure (>90 mmHg) dobutamine (inotropic) or levosimendan (inotropic/vasodilator) may be preferable. Noradrenaline (vasopressor) may be preferable in cardiogenic shock or septicaemia.

24. A. The clinical history suggests acute stent thrombosis. The image shows occlusion of flow at the proximal edge of a stent.

25. A. Current guidelines in the UK and Europe are 12 months dual-antiplatelet therapy (DAPT) after an acute coronary syndrome irrespective of the treatment or stent type. In elective angioplasty with a bare metal stent only 1 month of DAPT is required, followed by long-term aspirin as opposed to 12 months for drug-eluting stents (DESs). However, new-generation DESs with biocompatible or biodegradable polymers (the delivery agent for the drug) are showing safety with shorter durations, down to 3 months in some cases.

VALVULAR HEART DISEASE AND ENDOCARDITIS

1. **You review a 59-year-old man with long-standing hypertension in clinic. He has no other comorbidities. He complains of some breathlessness, but this does not limit his physical activity. A transthoracic echocardiogram demonstrates aortic root dilatation and severe aortic regurgitation.**

   Which one of the following is not an indication for surgery?

   A. NYHA class II breathlessness
   B. Aortic root disease with maximal diameter 49 mm
   C. Patients undergoing CABG, valve surgery, or surgery of the ascending aorta
   D. Asymptomatic with resting LVEF ≤50%
   E. Asymptomatic with end-diastolic dimension > 70 mm

2. **You are asked to review the echocardiogram of a 74-year-old woman with a loud pansystolic murmur (📹 Video 3.1).**

   The following statements are all true, except:

   A. The jet of regurgitation is anteriorly directed
   B. The regurgitation is likely to be chronic
   C. Using PISA to assess the severity of the regurgitant jet is more accurate than measuring the vena contracta
   D. The MV inflow E-wave velocity is 1.6 m/s; this suggests severe MR
   E. Systolic pulmonary vein flow reversal is not a sensitive measure of severe MR

3. You are reviewing a 65-year-old farmer in the post-PCI clinic. He had primary angioplasty to his **RCA** for an inferior **STEMI** 3 months previously. He reports exertional breathlessness but no chest pain. His current medications are aspirin 75 mg od, clopidogrel 75 mg od, ramipril 5 mg bd, bisoprolol 5 mg od, and atorvastatin 80 mg od. On examination his **BP** is 110/70 mmHg and his heart rate is 60 bpm. You hear a soft pan-systolic murmur at his apex. His chest is clear and there is no pedal oedema. His **ECG** shows atrial fibrillation. He manages only 3 minutes on the treadmill with no chest pain or **ECG** changes, stopping due to breathlessness. You request an urgent echocardiogram, which demonstrates mild **LV** systolic dysfunction. The inferior wall is akinetic, there is some tethering of the posterior mitral valve leaflet, and as a result some mitral regurgitation (**ERO = 0.2 cm²**).

   What is the next appropriate step in his management?

   A. Start dabigatran
   B. Start eplerenone
   C. Urgent repeat coronary angiography
   D. Discharge patient with reassurance that he has reasonable LV function and no significant valve disease
   E. Stress echocardiography

4. An 82-year-old retired solicitor presents to the **ED** with chest pain radiating to his jaw. He has hypertension treated with ramipril 5 mg bd but is otherwise normally fit and well. His admission **ECG** shows atrial fibrillation with a ventricular rate of 90 bpm, **LVH**, and widespread **ST** segment depression. His peak troponin is 110 ng/L (normal <30 ng/L). He is started on treatment for an acute coronary syndrome and listed for an inpatient angiogram. You are asked to perform a bedside echocardiogram as a systolic murmur is heard on the post-take ward round.

   Calculate the aortic valve area (using the continuity equation) from Figures 3.1–3.3.

   A. 0.76 cm²
   B. 0.80 cm²
   C. 0.92 cm²
   D. 1.02 cm²
   E. 1.08 cm²

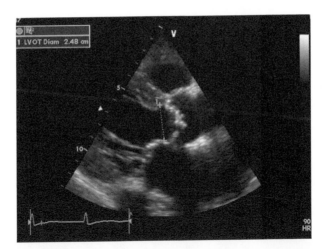

Figure 3.1

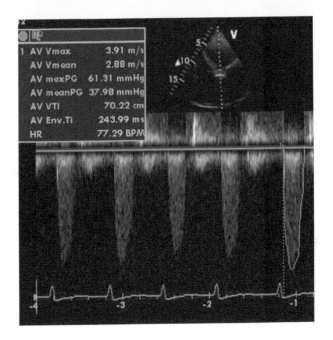

Figure 3.2

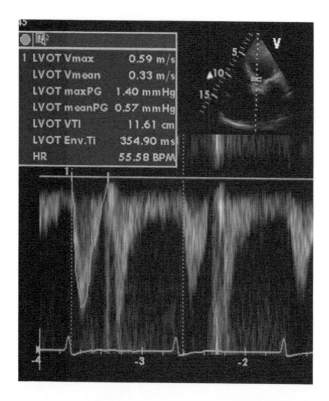

Figure 3.3

5. **The patient in Question 4 goes on to have a coronary angiogram. It shows:**

    - LMS: mild atheroma
    - LAD: severe (90%) proximal stenosis; good distal target
    - LCx: small vessel with diffuse distal atheroma
    - RCA: dominant; moderate (50–60%) mid-vessel focal stenosis.

    Which one of the following statements is correct?

    A. The patient should be referred for AVR and LIMA to LAD
    B. His operative mortality is about 3%
    C. Surgical ablation for AF may be considered
    D. The patient should have PCI to LAD followed by TAVI
    E. He should be managed conservatively with a beta-blocker and warfarin

6. **A 68-year-old man is referred for assessment of an ejection
    systolic murmur after presenting with worsening breathlessness.
    Image loops taken from his transthoracic echocardiogram
    are shown in ▣ Video 3.2 and ▣ Video 3.3. The following
    measurements were obtained during transthoracic echo:**

    - mean gradient across aortic valve, 30 mmHg
    - aortic valve area (by continuity equation), 1.0 cm²

    **Coronary angiography demonstrated mild atheroma without any
    significant disease.**

    Which one of the following would be the most useful next investigation?

    A. Repeat transthoracic echocardiogram in 6 months
    B. Transoesophageal echocardiography
    C. Dobutamine stress echocardiography
    D. Exercise tolerance test for risk stratification
    E. Repeat transthoracic echocardiogram in 12 months

7. **A 79-year-old retired farmer with known aortic stenosis (AS)
    returns for his annual surveillance echocardiogram. He remains
    physically active with no symptoms. His BP is 180/110 mmHg.**

    The following summary is obtained:

    - Severe AS—peak velocity has increased from 3.8 m/s a year ago to 4.0 m/s today
    - Mean gradient, 40 mmHg
    - Aortic valve area, 1.0 cm²
    - Mild LVH
    - Good overall LV systolic function

    Which one of the following statements is correct?

    A. A statin should be prescribed to reduce the rate of AS progression
    B. An antihypertensive drug should be prescribed
    C. The increase in peak velocity of ≥0.2 m/s/year suggests that surgery should be considered
    D. An exercise tolerance test (ETT) is unsafe in asymptomatic severe AS
    E. An elevated BNP of 120 pg/ml suggests that surgery should be considered

8. **Three years later, the patient in Question 5 is admitted to hospital with chest pain. A repeat echocardiogram shows a heavily calcified aortic valve with a peak velocity of 4.8 m/s, valve area of 0.8 cm², and moderately impaired LV systolic function. Two years ago he had a right upper lobe lung lobectomy with chemoradiotherapy for a localized primary bronchogenic carcinoma. Your consultant has asked you to write a referral letter to the 'heart team' at the regional tertiary centre to consider this patient for a transcatheter aortic valve implantation (TAVI).**

   Which one of the following is a contraindication for TAVI?

   A. Plaques with mobile thrombi in the ascending aorta or arch
   B. Porcelain aorta
   C. Home oxygen therapy
   D. Severe peripheral vascular disease
   E. LVEF <30%

9. **The Doppler profile shown in Figure 3.4 is taken from a patient presenting with breathlessness.**

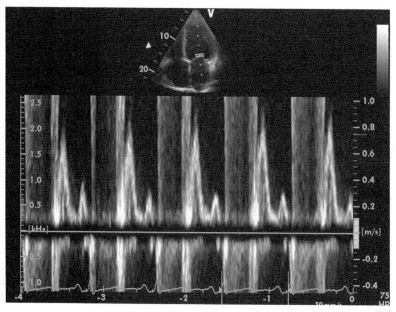

Figure 3.4

   What is this Doppler profile least likely to be compatible with?

   A. Chronic secondary mitral regurgitation
   B. Severe mitral stenosis
   C. Aortic stenosis with concentric LVH
   D. Cardiac amyloidosis
   E. Diastolic dysfuntion

10. **You are asked to review an echocardiogram of a 82-year-old woman who has both severe aortic stenosis (AS) and severe mitral regurgitation (MR).**

    All the following statements are true in patients with combined or multiple valve lesions except:

    A. Associated MR may lead to underestimation of the severity of AS

    B. Severe AS may lead to overestimation of coexisting MR

    C. Significant aortic regurgitation (AR) lengthens the Doppler pressure half-time (PHT) in mitral stenosis (MS)

    D. The presence of significant AR may overestimate the gradient across the aortic valve

    E. Planimetry should be utlilized

11. **A 24-year-old IV drug user presents to hospital with a 6-week history of fever, rigors, and general malaise. On admission his temperature is 38°C. His venous pressure is elevated to the angle of the jaw with prominent V waves. You hear a loud systolic murmur at the lower left sternal edge, which is louder on inspiration. There is mild pedal oedema. Blood cultures grow *Staphylococcus aureus* in all six bottles. An initial transthoracic echocardiogram followed by a transoesophageal echocardiogram show no obvious vegetation and severe tricuspid regurgitation (TR). Nonetheless, he has 6 weeks of intravenous antibiotics with resolution of his sepsis. There are no embolic complications. He is now asymptomatic.**

    The following are all appropriate considerations for tricuspid valve surgery except:

    A. Persistent symptoms with reasonable right ventricular dysfunction

    B. No symptoms—TAPSE 12 mm

    C. No symptoms—tricuspid annulus systolic velocity 13 cm/s

    D. No symptoms—RV end-systolic area 30 cm²

    E. All the above are appropriate indications for surgery

12. **Which one of the following transthoracic echocardiographic parameters does not suggest severe aortic regurgitation?**

    A. Vena contracta 0.50 cm

    B. Central jet width 70% of LVOT

    C. Holodiastolic aortic flow reversal in descending aorta

    D. Pressure half-time 190 ms

    E. Effective regurgitant orifice area ≥ 0.3 cm²

13. **During your CCU ward round you review a 72-year-old man with known aortic stenosis who presented with angina. He has been referred for aortic valve replacement. He has heard that there are different types of valve replacement and asks which is best.**

    Which one of the following statements is false?

    A. A mechanical prosthesis is preferred for patients with hyperparathyroidism
    B. Patient lifestyle is an important factor in decision-making
    C. A bioprosthetic valve is preferred for patients with limited life expectancy
    D. A bioprosthetic valve is preferred for young women contemplating pregnancy
    E. Bioprosthetic valves are preferred for patients who have previously undergone CABG

14. **A 23-year-old man with transposition of the great arteries underwent a Mustard operation during childhood. Three months previously he had a stent for a baffle stenosis. He attends outpatient clinic. He is undergoing a root canal procedure the following week and his dental surgeon has asked whether he needs prophylaxis for infective endocarditis (IE) before the procedure. He has a history of penicillin allergy.**

    What would you recommend?

    A. No antibiotic prophylaxis required
    B. IV oxacillin 2 g 60 minutes before the procedure
    C. Oral amoxicillin 1 g 30 minutes before the procedure with steroid and antihistamine
    D. IV cephalexin 2 g 60 minutes before the procedure
    E. IV/oral clindamycin 600 mg 30 minutes before the procedure

15. **A 38-year-old IV drug abuser presents with a 1-week history of malaise, fatigue, and rigors. His temperature on admission was 38.5°C. Examination revealed a pan-systolic murmur which was loudest at the left sternal edge. Three sets of blood cultures were taken. Transthoracic echocardiography (TTE) showed vegetation on the tricuspid valve with moderate TR.**

    Which one of the following organisms is most likely to be positive in blood cultures?

    A. *Streptococcus sanguis*
    B. *Enterococcus faecium*
    C. *Coxiella burnetii*
    D. *Staphylococcus aureus*
    E. *Kingella kingae*

16. **A 76-year-old man presents to the ED with a 2-week history of fever, chills, poor appetite, and weight loss. He had a bovine aortic valve replacement 5 years previously for severe aortic stenosis. He was pyrexial. Admission bloods revealed a white cell count of 16.0 × 10⁹/L and C-reactive protein (CRP) 120 mg/dL. TOE was performed the next day (see 🎞 Video 3.4).**

    What is the abnormality shown on the echocardiogram?

    A. Vegetation on the aortic valve
    B. Aortic root abscess
    C. Vegetation on the anterior mitral leaflet
    D. Severe central mitral regurgitation
    E. Severe tricuspid regurgitation

17. **A 59-year-old man with a bicuspid aortic valve and a background of benign prostatic hypertrophy presents with a 1-week history of fever and lethargy. He had been treated by his GP with oral antibiotics for a urinary tract infection (UTI) a week prior to admission. On examination, an ejection systolic murmur was audible on auscultation. As part of his initial investigations routine bloods and blood and urine cultures were taken. His urine culture sent by his GP has grown *Escherichia coli*. The admitting team suspects endocarditis.**

    What is the next step of management?

    A. Treat UTI with different antibiotics than those used previously
    B. Arrange a transthoracic echocardiogram (TTE).
    C. Arrange a transoesophageal echocardiogram (TOE) as aortic valve vegetations are poorly visualized on TTE
    D. Repeat urine culture
    E. Arrange cardiac MRI to rule out endocarditis

18. **Which one of the following is a predictor of poor outcome in patients with infective endocarditis?**

    A. Insulin-dependent diabetes mellitus
    B. Renal failure
    C. Echocardiographic evidence of peri-annular complications
    D. *Staphylococcus aureus* in blood cultures
    E. All the above

19. **An 80-year-old woman with a background of moderate aortic stenosis presents with a 2-week history of fatigue, weight loss, and night sweats. She has a history of nausea and altered bowel habit. Bloods revealed Hb 9.9 g/dL, white cell count 16.0 × 10⁹/L, and CRP 187 mg/L. Blood cultures were taken on admission and she was commenced on empirical antibiotics. TTE demonstrated an aortic valve vegetation.**

    The presence of which one of the following organisms would prompt gastrointestinal investigations?

    A. *Haemophilus para-influenzae*
    B. *Cardiobacterium hominis*
    C. *Streptococcus bovis*
    D. *Enterococcus faecalis*
    E. Coagulase-negative staphylococci

20. **A 71-year-old man presents 10 months after aortic valve replacement with fatigue, weight loss, and fever. Six weeks previously he had had treatment for a dental abscess. Whilst results from blood culture were awaited, a transthoracic echocardiogram revealed an aortic valve vegetation.**

    Which of the following is the most appropriate next step?

    A. Start vancomycin with gentamicin and rifampicin
    B. Arrange urgent TEE
    C. Wait for identification and sensitivities of cultures
    D. Repeat TTE in 1 week
    E. Start amoxicillin plus clavulanic acid and gentamycin, and arrange urgent TTE

21. **A 51-year-old farmer presents with low-grade fever and a recent history of weight loss. He has been investigated by his GP and general physicians but no cause has been identified for his symptoms. His inflammatory markers are raised and a TTE shows a 0.5 × 0.3 cm echogenic mass attached to the non-coronary cusp of the aortic valve. Endocarditis is suspected, although multiple blood cultures are negative.**

    Which one of the following organisms is the most likely cause of persistently negative cultures?

    A. *Streptococcus constellatus*
    B. Coagulase-negative staphylococci
    C. *Cardiobacterium hominis*
    D. *Streptococus sanguis*
    E. *Coxiella burnetii*

22. **Which one of the following statements regarding outpatient parenteral antibiotic therapy (OPAT) for infective endocarditis is true?**

    A. OPAT can be considered in oral-streptococci-positive endocarditis in stable patients with no complications in the critical phase (0–2 weeks)

    B. Complications are rare in the first 2 weeks

    C. OPAT in patients who have received inpatient therapy for 3 weeks can be considered despite the presence of heart failure

    D. Daily post-discharge evaluation physician review is necessary for OPAT

    E. Neurological features are not a contraindication to OPAT

1. B. This man's echocardiogram shows a dilated aortic root. In this case the likely cause is his long-standing hypertension. In aortic root disease indication for surgery is based on the maximal aortic diameter, regardless of the severity of aortic regurgitation. Patients with Marfan's syndrome should be offered surgery when their aortic root diameter is ≥45 mm; the figure is ≥50 mm for patients with a bicuspid aortic valve and ≥55 mm for any other patient (including those with aortic root dilatation secondary to hypertension, as in this case). Other indications for surgery in severe aortic regurgitation are:

- Symptomatic patients (NYHA class II, III, or IV dyspnoea or angina)
- Asymptomatic patients with resting LVEF ≤50%
- Patients undergoing CABG, valve surgery, or surgery of the ascending aorta.
- Asymptomatic patients with resting LVEF >50% with severe LV dilatation—LV end-diastolic dimension >70 mm or LV end-systolic dimension >50 mm (or >25 mm/m² BSA).

2. C. The video shows prolapse of the posterior mitral valve leaflet. There is eccentric MR. The vena contracta (VC) can be measured in both central and eccentric jets to estimate the severity of MR. The VC should ideally be measured in the apical four-chamber view. PISA is more accurate for central regurgitant jets. Systolic pulmonary vein flow reversal is specific for severe MR, but is not sensitive. Echocardiographic criteria for the definition of severe mitral regurgitation are shown in Table 3.1.

Table 3.1 ESC guidelines 2012

Valve morphology	Flail leaflet/rupture papillary muscle/large coaptation defect
Colour flow regurgitant jet	Very large central jet or eccentric jet adhering, swirling, and reaching the posterior wall of the LA
CW signal of regurgitant jet	Dense/triangular
Other qualitative measure	Large flow convergence zone
Vena contracta	≥7 mm (>8 mm for biplane)
Upstream vein flow	Systolic pulmonary vein flow reversal
MV inflow	E-wave dominant ≥1.5 m/s
Other semi-quantitative measure	TVI mitral/TVI aortic >1.4
ERO (mm²)	≥40 (primary), ≥20 (secondary)
Regurgitant volume (mL/beat)	≥60 (primary), ≥30 (secondary)
Enlargement of cardiac chambers	LV, LA

Reproduced from 'Guidelines on the management of valvular heart disease', *Eur Heart J*, 2012; **33**: 2451–96, with permission of Oxford University Press.

3. E. This patient has secondary MR. His recent infarct has led to alteration of his LV geometry (inferior akinesis) resulting in tethering of structurally normal MV leaflets. Ischaemic MR is a dynamic condition and its severity may vary depending upon changes in loading conditions.

The ESC Guidelines published in 2012 propose that, because of their prognostic value, lower thresholds of severity using quantitative methods should be used in secondary MR. An ERO ≥ 20 mm^2 or a regurgitant volume ≥ 30 mL/beat suggests severe MR.

As ischaemic MR is a dynamic condition, stress testing may play a role in its evaluation. An exercise-induced increase in the ERO of ≥ 13 mm^2 has been shown to be associated with a large increase in the relative risk of death and hospitalization for cardiac decompensation (ESC Guidelines 2012).

4. B.

$$CSA_{AV} = CSA_{LVOT} \times VTI_{LVOT}/VTI_{AV}$$
$$CSA_{LVOT} = 0.785(2.48^2)$$
$$CSA_{AV} = 4.82 \times 11.61/70.22$$
$$CSA_{AV} = 0.798 \text{ cm}^2 = 0.8 \text{ cm}^2$$

5. C. This patient has severe symptomatic aortic stenosis and two moderate to severe coronary stenoses with good distal targets. As he has no other significant comorbidity, he should be referred for AVR and two-vessel CABG. PCI and TAVI should be considered only if the patient is judged to be unsuitable for AVR after surgical consultation. In patients with a primary indication for aortic/mitral valve surgery, CABG is recommended for coronary artery stenosis $\geq 70\%$ and should be considered for coronary artery stenosis ≥ 50–70% (ESC Guidelines 2012).

This patient's operative mortality for AVR and CABG is likely to be at least 4.5%. Table 3.2 shows the estimated operative mortality after surgery for valvular heart disease. AF is an independent risk factor for poor outcome after cardiac surgery. The ESC Guidelines for the management of AF recommend that surgical ablation should be considered in patients with symptomatic AF and may be performed in patients with asymptomatic AF undergoing cardiac surgery if feasible with minimal risk.

Table 3.2 ESC guidelines 2012: operative mortality after surgery for valvular heart disease

	EACTS (2010)	STS (2010)*	UK (2004–2008)	Germany (2009)
Aortic valve replacement, no CABG (%)	2.9 (40 662)	3.7 (25 515)	2.8 (17 636)	2.9 (11 981)
Aortic valve replacement	5.5 (24 890)	4.5 (18 227)	5.3 (12 491)	6.1 (9113)
Mitral valve repair, no CABG (%)	2.1 (3231)	1.6 (7293)	2 (3283)	2 (3335)
Mitral valve replacement, no CABG (%)	4.3 (6838)	6.0 (5448)	6.1 (3614)	7.8 (1855)
Mitral valve repair/ replacement + CABG (%)	6.8/11.4 (2515/1612)	4.6/11.1 (4721/2427)	8.3/11.1 (2021/1337)	6.5/14.5 (1785/837)

*Mortality for STS includes first and redo interventions.

The number of patients is given in parentheses

EACTS, European Association for Cardiothoracic Surgery; STS, Society of Thoracic Surgeons (USA).

Reproduced from 'Guidelines on the management of valvular heart disease', *Eur Heart J*, 2012; **33**: 2451–96, with permission of Oxford University Press.

6. C. This patient has a small aortic valve area and a modest peak gradient in the context of LV impairment (low flow, low gradient AS). In this subset of individuals low-dose dobutamine stress echocardiography can help to distinguish truly severe AS from pseudo-severe AS.

- True AS: there would be little change in valve area (<0.2 cm² and remaining <1.1 cm²) but a significant increase in aortic valve gradients
- Pseudo-severe AS: the valve area becomes bigger.

7. B. There is no good evidence from randomized controlled trials that statins affect the progression of AS. Exercise testing is contraindicated in symptomatic patients with AS but is recommended in physically active patients for unmasking symptoms and in the risk stratification of asymptomatic patients with severe AS. The development of symptoms or a fall in blood pressure is a predictor of symptom development/poor outcome and therefore is an indication for surgery (ESC Guidelines 2012). In addition, the guidelines recommend that if patients are not physically active or exercise testing is negative, surgery should or may be considered in the presence of specific risk factors and low/intermediate individual surgical risk. These risk factors are shown in Box 3.1.

Box 3.1 Risk factors for consideration of aortic valve surgery
Peak velocity >5.5 m/s
Severe valve calcification + peak velocity progression ≥0.3 m/s/year
Markedly elevated natriuretic peptide levels
Mean gradient increase with exercise >20 mmHg
Excessive LV hypertrophy without a history of hypertension

A BNP level of 120 pg/mL is only mildly elevated and may be due to other causes. A very raised BNP level is defined as >400 pg/mL.

8. A. TAVI is recommended for patients with symptomatic severe AS who, according to the 'heart team', are unsuitable for conventional surgery because of severe comorbidity. Various factors need to be taken into account when making this assessment. A logistic Euro-SCORE of ≥20% has been suggested as an indication for TAVI therapy, but in patients with a lower Euro-SCORE other conditions such as a porcelain aorta, a history of chest radiation, and patent coronary bypass grafts make AVR less suitable.

Specific contraindications for TAVI that are listed in Table 3.3.

9. B. The E:A ratio is >2 with a deceleration time of <150 ms in keeping with severe diastolic dysfunction. Assessment of the severity of mitral stenosis using pressure half-time (PHT) should be performed with continuous-wave (CW) Doppler. The PHT in severe MR is long (>220 ms). The mitral valve area can be calculated using the formula MVA = 220/PHT. Although the Doppler trace shown in Figure 3.4 is a pulsed wave (PW) of LV inflow. It would be unusual to obtain this pattern in severe MS.

Table 3.3 ESC Guidelines 2012: contraindications for transcather aortic valve implantatation (TAVI)

Absolute contraindications

Absence of a 'heart team' and no cardiac surgery on the site

Appropriateness of TAVI, as an alternative toAVR, not confirmed by a 'heart team'

Clinical

Estimated life expectancy <1 year

Improvement of quality of life by TAVI unlikely because of comorbidities

Severe primary associated disease of other valves, with major contribution to the patient's symptoms, which can only be treated by surgery

Anatomical

Inadequate annulus size (<18 mm, >29 mm^2)

Thrombus in the left ventricle

Active endocarditis

Elevated risk of coronary ostium obstruction (asymmetric valve calcification, short distance between annulus and coronary ostium, small aortic sinuses)

Plaques with mobile thrombi in the ascending aorta or arch

For transfemoral/subclavian approach: inadequate vascular access (vessel size, calcification, tortuosity)

Relative contraindications

Bicuspid or non-calcified valves

Untreated coronary artery disease requiring revascularization

Haemodynamic instability

LVEF <20%

For transapical approach: severe pulmonary disease, LV apex not accessible

Reproduced from 'Guidelines on the management of valvular heart disease', *Eur Heart J*, 2012; **33**: 2451–96, with permission of Oxford University Press.

10. C. AR shortens the PHT in mitral stenosis. PHT is a measure of the change in pressure between two cardiac chambers. In significant AR, there is likely to be high LV end-diastolic pressures. This leads to a higher pressure difference between the LV and LA—hence shortening of the PHT in MS. This underestimates the severity of MS.

Associated MR leads to underestimation of the severity of AS since decreased stroke volume due to MR lowers the flow (and gradient) across the AV. Similarly, severe AS causes high ventricular pressures leading to overestimation of coexistent MR

In mixed aortic valve disease, the presence of significant AR will lead to increased stroke volume and hence flow (and gradient) across the aortic valve. Therefore AR can overestimate the severity of AS.

Methods that are less dependent on loading conditions, such as planimetry of valve area, should be utilized.

11. C. This patient has severe isolated primary tricuspid regurgitation. Indications for surgery are shown in Box 3.2. Evaluation of RV dimensions and function must be conducted. Patients with RV dysfunction can be identified by various indices including a TAPSE (<15 mm), tricuspid annular systolic velocity <11 cm/s, and RV end-systolic area >20 cm^2.

Box 3.2 ESC Guidelines 2012

Surgery is indicated in symptomatic patients without severe RV dysfunction. In patients undergoing left-sided valve surgery, tricuspid valve surgery should be considered for moderate primary TR or mild–moderate secondary TR with dilated annulus (≥40 mm or ≥21 mm/m^2). Surgery should also be considered in asymptomatic or mildly symptomatic patients with severe isolated primary TR and progressive RV dilatation or deterioration of right ventricular function.

Adapted from 'Guidelines on the management of valvular heart disease', *Eur Heart J*, 2012; **33**: 2451–96, with permission of Oxford University Press.

---

12. A. The following parameters suggest severe aortic regurgitation:
- Central jet width >65% of LVOT
- Vena contracta >0.6 cm
- Pressure half time <200 ms
- Holodiastolic aortic flow reversal in descending aorta
- Moderate or greater LV enlargement (BSE guidelines for chamber quantification give 6.4 cm as the lower limit of moderate LV diastolic enlargement in men)
- Regurgitant volume ≥ 60 mL/beat
- Regurgitant fraction ≥50%
- Effective regurgitant orifice area ≥0.3 cm^2.

13. E. A mechanical valve is preferred in patients for whom redo valve surgery would be high risk (LV dysfunction, previous CABG, multiple valve prosthesis). Any valve replacement carries risk, and in deciding whether a mechanical or biological valve is best a number of factors should be considered. The choice is mainly determined by estimating the risk of anticoagulant-related bleeding and thromboembolism with a mechanical valve compared with the risk of structural valve deterioration with a bioprosthesis. The ESC Guidelines 2012 are as follows.

In favour of mechanical prosthesis:
- Desire of the informed patient and absence of contraindication for long-term anticoagulation
- Patients at risk of accelerated structural valve deterioration, including young age (<40 years) and hyperparathyroidism
- Patients already on anticoagulation because of other mechanical prostheses
- Patients already on anticoagulation because at high risk for thromboembolism
- Age <60 years (aortic prosthesis) and <65 years (mitral prosthesis). In patients aged 60–65 years who receive an aortic prosthesis and those between 65 and 70 years in the case of mitral prosthesis, both valves are acceptable and the choice requires careful analysis of factors other than age
- Patients with a reasonable life expectancy (>10 years), for whom future redo valve surgery would be high risk.

In favour of bioprosthesis:

- Desire of the informed patient
- Unavailability of good-quality anticoagulation (contraindication or high risk, unwillingness, compliance problems, lifestyle, occupation)
- Reoperation for mechanical valve thrombosis despite good long-term anticoagulant control
- Patients for whom future redo valve surgery would be low risk
- Limited life expectancy (lower than the presumed durability of the bioprosthesis), or age >65 years (aortic prosthesis) or >70 years (mitral prosthesis)
- Young women contemplating pregnancy.

14. E.   According to ESC guidelines, antibiotic prophylaxis is considered for those at highest risk for infective endocarditis (e.g. prosthetic valve, previous endocarditis, cyanotic congenital heart disease, or congenital heart disease with complete repair and with prosthetic material insertion within the last 6 months or if there is a residual defect after a repair with prosthetic material), those are undergoing high-risk procedures (dental procedures involving perforation of oral mucosa or manipulation of the gingiva or the periapical region of the teeth). Antibiotic prophylaxis is no longer recommended for other procedures. Cephalosporins should not be used in patients who have had anaphylaxis, angio-oedema, or urticaria due to use of penicillin and ampicillin.

15. D.   Approximately 85% of IE cases are culture-positive. *Staphylococcus aureus* is the most common cause in IV drug abusers. The HACEK group is the most common cause of culture-negative endocarditis. Candida endocarditis is a severe manifestation of systemic candidiasis and is the most common cause of fungal IE.

16. B.   The transoesophageal echocardiogram shows the long-axis view which includes the aortic and mitral valves. The translucent area above the aortic valve replacement is an aortic root abscess. There is severe paravalvular aoric regurgitation. In addition colour flow is seen between the aortic root and the left atrium (superior to the anterior mitral valve leaflet) which represents a perforation of the anterior mitral valve leaflet/annulus attachment.

17. B.   According to ESC Guidelines 2009, TTE is the first-line imaging modality in cases of suspected endocarditis. TOE should be done if suspicion of IE is high and TTE is normal or inconclusive.

18. E.   The in-hospital mortality rate of patients with IE varies from 9.6% to 26%, but differs considerably from patient to patient. Prognosis in IE is influenced by four main factors: patient characteristics, the presence or absence of cardiac and non-cardiac complications, the infecting organism, and echocardiographic findings. The risk of patients with left-sided IE has been formally assessed according to these variables. Patients with heart failure, periannular complications, and/or *Staphylococcus aureus* infection are at highest risk of death and need for surgery in the active phase of the disease. When three of these factors are present, the risk reaches 79%. A high degree of comorbidity, insulin-dependent diabetes, depressed left ventricular function, and the presence of stroke are also predictors of poor in-hospital outcome. In those patients who need urgent surgery, persistent infection and renal failure are predictors of mortality. Predictably, patients with an indication for surgery who cannot proceed owing to prohibitive surgical risk have the worst prognosis.

19. C. Group D streptococci (*Streptococcus bovis*) are an increasingly frequent cause of IE, especially in the elderly, and are associated with colonic disease.

20. A. First-line empirical antibiotic treatment for endocarditis which occurs <12 months post-surgery is a combination of vancomycin, gentamycin, and rifampicin.

21. E. Infective endocarditis associated with constantly negative blood cultures can be caused by intracellular bacteria such as *Coxiella burnetii, Bartonella, Chlamydia*, and, as recently demonstrated, *Tropheryma whipplei*. These account for up to 5% of all IE. Diagnosis in such cases relies on serological testing, cell culture, or gene amplification. The HACEK group (*Haemophilus parainfluenzae, H.aphrophilus, H.paraphrophilus, H.influenzae, Actinobacillus actinomycetemcomitans, Cardiobacterium hominis, Eikenella corrodens, Kingella kingae*, and *K.denitrificans*), *Brucella*, fungi, and nutritionally variant streptococci may also cause infective endocarditis that is frequently associated with negative blood cultures.

22. A. The following criteria determine the suitability of outpatient parenteral antibiotic therapy (OPAT) for infective endocarditis.

- Critical phase (0–2 weeks): complications occur during this phase; inpatient treatment preferable during this phase; consider OPAT if oral streptococci, patient is stable, and no complications
- Continuation phase (beyond week 2): consider OPAT if medically stable. Do not consider OPAT if heart failure is present or there are concerning echocardiographic features, neurological signs, or renal impairment. Regular post-discharge evaluation is possible (nurse, once daily; physician in charge, once or twice weekly).

1. **A 55-year-old man with known heart failure and LVEF of 37% is reviewed in the outpatient clinic with breathlessness. He is NYHA class III with no signs of fluid overload on examination. His BP is 110/60 mmHg, and his heart rate is 55 bpm. He is on bisoprolol 5 mg od and ramipril 10 mg od. His U&E tests reveal Na 137 mmol/L, K 4.5 mmol/L, urea 7 mmol/L, and creatinine 85 μmol/L.**

   Which one of the following medications will you chose next?

   A. Furosemide 40 mg od
   B. Spironolactone 25 mg od
   C. Digoxin 62.5 micrograms od
   D. Hydralazine 37.5 mg and isosorbide dinitrate 20 mg od
   E. Candesartan 4 mg od

2. **An 80-year-old woman is admitted with acute pulmonary oedema on a background of progressive shortness of breath with exertional chest pain for 6 months. She has a history of renal impairment with an eGFR of 40 mL/min. She is initially commenced on IV furosemide with good effect. An echocardiogram reveals LVEF 40% with severe aortic stenosis (AS) with an estimated valve area of 0.7 cm².**

   What would you do next?

   A. Add a beta-blocker
   B. Perform angiography with a view to aortic valve replacement (AVR)/transcatheter aortic valve implantation
   C. Add an ACE inhibitor
   D. Implant a CRT-D
   E. A and B

3. **You review a 60-year-old man with NHYA class II heart failure in clinic. He has LVEF 35%, BP 110/50 mmHg, and heart rate 80 bpm (sinus rhythm). Current medications are bisoprolol 1.25 mg and ramipril 7.5mg.**

    What medication alteration would you recommend to the GP?

    A. Add ivabradine
    B. Add spironolactone 25 mg od
    C. Add digoxin 62.5 micrograms od
    D. Titrate up bisoprolol
    E. Add candesartan 4 mg

4. **A 35-year-old man presents to the medical take with acute heart failure. He has a 2-week history of progressive breathlessness. Past medical history includes type II diabetes mellitus. An echocardiogram subsequently shows an EF of 25% with anterior, septal, and lateral wall motion defects. He is stabilized on medication with furosemide, spironolactone, bisoprolol, and ramipril.**

    What would be your next course of investigation?

    A. Endomyocardial biopsy
    B. Angiogram
    C. Viral titres
    D. Exercise tolerance test
    E. Lung function tests

5. **A 65-year-old woman with ischaemic cardiomyopathy and LVEF 30% comes for review in the outpatient clinic. She is NYHA class II and has been optimally revascularized. Her current heart failure medications are bisoprolol 10 mg od, ramipril 10 mg od, ivabradine 7.5 mg bd, and spironolactone 25 mg. Her ECG shows sinus rhythm, left bundle branch block (QRS duration 135 ms), left axis deviation, and PR interval 180 ms.**

    Which one of the following managements would you recommend next?

    A. Refer for transplant assessment
    B. Refer for ICD
    C. Refer for CRT-D
    D. Refer for CRT-P
    E. Perform a dyssynchrony echocardiogram

6. **A 65-year-old man presents to the chest pain clinic with a 2-month history of exertional chest pain. He has no past medical history of note. On examination his BP is 130/70 mmHg and his heart rate is 65 bpm in sinus rhythm with a 3/6 pansystolic murmur. He has a positive ETT with inferolateral ST segment depression at 5 minutes Bruce protocol. Coronary angiography reveals severe distal left main stem disease, severe mid-LAD disease, severe mid-circumflex disease, and severe distal RCA disease. An echocardiogram shows severe mitral regurgitation with moderate LV systolic dysfunction. CMR confirms viability in all territories.**

   What should you do next?

   A. Refer for multi-vessel angioplasty
   B. Continue medical management
   C. Refer for CABG
   D. Refer for mitral valve repair/replacement
   E. C and D

7. **You get a phone call from the heart failure nurse specialist regarding a patient followed up in clinic for titration of medication. He has dilated cardiomyopathy with an EF of 30%. His most recent BP is 110/60 mmHg with heart rate 60 bpm. He is currently on bisoprolol 7.5 mg od and ramipril 5 mg od. His renal function test results have been phoned through to the specialist nurse: Na 136 mmol/L, K 5.5 mmol/L, urea 13 mmol/L, creatinine 270 μmol/L. (Baseline before titration of ACE inhibitor: Na 138 mmol/L, K 4.8 mmol/L, urea 8 mmol/L, creatinine 180 μmol/L.)**

   What would be your advice?

   A. Continue current medication and recheck U&E at 1 week
   B. Stop ramipril and recheck U&E at 1 week
   C. Add spironolactone and recheck U&E at 1 week
   D. Halve dose of ramipril and recheck U&E at 1 week
   E. Stop all medication and recheck U&E at 1 week

8. **A 36-year-old woman with known idiopathic dilated cardiomyopathy (confirmed by TTE and angiography) is reviewed in the heart failure clinic. She is NYHA class III. Her current medication is bisoprolol 10 mg od, ramipril 7.5 mg od, spironolactone 25 mg od, digoxin 62.5 micrograms od, furosemide 40 mg bd. She has CRT-D *in situ*. Her heart rate is 70 bpm and her BP is 85/40 mmHg. She has mild peripheral oedema and a raised JVP.**

   What is your next step?

   A. Add candesartan 8 mg od
   B. Perform CMR
   C. Refer for transplant assessment
   D. Increase ramipril
   E. Stop ramipril and furosemide

9. **A 57-year-old woman with known heart failure and EF 42% is reviewed in clinic. She is breathless on walking up one flight of stairs or half a mile on the flat. On examination, her BP is 130/90 mmHg and her heart rate is 75 bpm (SR, ECG QRS < 120 ms). Her chest is clear to auscultation. There are no signs of fluid overload. Her current medication is carvedilol 25 mg bd, furosemide 40 mg od, and digoxin 62.5 micrograms od. Her recent renal function tests are Na 141 mmol/L, K 5.1 mmol/L, urea 13.5 mmol/L, and creatinine 236 µmol/L. She has not previously tolerated an ACE inhibitor or spironolactone because of deteriorating renal function and hyperkalaemia.**

   What would you do next?

   A. Add hydralazine and isosorbide dinitrate (H-ISDN)
   B. Add candesartan
   C. Add eplerenone
   D. Add furosemide
   E. Add ivabradine

10. **A 30-year-old man had a cardiac transplant 5 years previously because of dilated cardiomyopathy. He initially did very well post-transplant. However, he has noticed that he is progressively short of breath on exertion. His TTE shows mid and apical anterior hypokinesia.**

    What is the most likely diagnosis?

    A. Acute T-cell rejection
    B. Non-Hodgkin's lymphoma
    C. Coronary vasculopathy
    D. Sarcoidosis
    E. None of the above

11. Which one of the following best describes the actions of ACE?

    A. Promotes the degradation of angiotensin II

    B. Directly stimulates the synthesis of aldosterone

    C. Stimulates the production of norepinephrine

    D. Converts angiotensin I to angiotensin II

    E. All of the above

12. A 55-year-old man presents with pulmonary oedema following an episode of chest pain a week previously. What does his CMR show (📹 Video 4.1)?

    A. Normal

    B. Global mild LV systolic dysfunction

    C. RWMA in the RCA territory with severe LVSD

    D. RWMA in the LAD territory with severe LVSD

    E. None of the above

13. Which one of the following is not a contraindication to an ACE inhibitor?

    A. History of angioedema

    B. Known renal artery stenosis

    C. TTE showing AVA 1.2 cm^2

    D. Serum creatinine 250 µmol/L

    E. Serum potassium 5.5 mmol/L

14. A 40-year-old man with known hypertrophic cardiomyopathy presents to the outpatient clinic with a history of increased breathlessness. He has noted a marked reduction in his exercise tolerance over the last 6 months and it is now limited to 100 yards despite his being commenced on bisoprolol. Clinical examination demonstrates a forceful apex and a mid-systolic murmur. There is no evidence of fluid overload. Echocardiography demonstrates asymmetric left ventricular hypertrophy with a septal thickness of 20 mm. There is a resting left ventricular outflow tract gradient of 60 mmHg.

What is the most appropriate management for this patient?

    A Dual-chamber pacing

    B ICD implantation

    C Referral for exercise stress echocardiography to assess for arrhythmia and increase in LVOT gradient

    D Change from bisoprolol to verapamil

    E Referral to a specialist centre for septal ablation

15. **A 25-year-old woman is referred with a mid-systolic murmur. Echocardiography demonstrates asymmetric left ventricular hypertrophy with good left ventricular systolic function. The septal thickness is 17 mm with a small left ventricular outflow tract gradient. She is symptom free.**

    Which one of the following statements is not true?

    A. A blood pressure response of <20 mmHg on standard exercise testing is a risk factor for sudden cardiac death

    B. First-degree relatives who have had normal screening echocardiograms should have repeat studies every 5 years

    C. The patient should be advised that future pregnancy is high risk

    D. She is at higher than normal risk of developing atrial fibrillation

    E. Beta-blocker therapy is not indicated

16. **A 53-year-old man presents to the outpatient clinic with symptoms of lethargy and tiredness. Clinical examination reveals him to be pale with a blood pressure of 110/70 mmHg, a JVP of +8 cmH$_2$O, and oedema to his mid-calf. His 12-lead ECG demonstrates a PR interval of 200 ms, a QRS duration of 145 ms, and poor R-wave progression. A subsequent echocardiogram was technically challenging, but demonstrated a thickened ventricle with a septal thickness of 15 mm. Overall systolic function is reported as normal. An E/A ratio was estimated to be 1.4 with tissue Doppler giving an E/E' ratio of 12.**

    Which one of the following investigations is most likely to help make the diagnosis?

    A. Myocardial biopsy

    B. Contrast-enhanced transthoracic echocardiogram

    C. Urine and serum electrophoresis for monoclonal protein

    D. Myocardial perfusion scan

    E. Left and right heart catheter

17. **A 73-year-old man well known to the ED with alcohol excess presented with acute pulmonary oedema requiring CPAP. His presenting ECG demonstrated sinus rhythm with a broad left bundle branch block with QRS duration of 173 ms. A subsequent coronary angiogram demonstrates the following:**

    LMS normal
    LAD 50% mid vessel stenosis
    LCx 60% distal stenosis
    RCA recessive vessel, 75% proximal disease

    A subsequent echocardiogram demonstrated a left ventricular diastolic dimension of 7 cm. There is global impairment of left ventricular systolic function with EF estimated at 30%. There was severe mitral regurgitation due to annular dilatation. He was successfully commenced on ramipril and bisoprolol.

    What is the most appropriate management at this stage?

    A. Referral for CRT-D
    B. Referral for revascularization
    C. Commence warfarin therapy for a dilated left ventricle
    D. Commence spironalactone
    E. Advise abstinence from alcohol and repeat echocardiogram at 6 weeks

18. **A 74-year-old patient presents to hospital with a VF arrest. She is successfully resuscitated and a subsequent ECG demonstrates a clear-cut anterior myocardial infarction with >2 mm ST elevation in leads V2–V6. Coronary angiography demonstrates a suboccluded proximal LAD, with a small unobstructed circumflex artery and a 70% stenosis in the proximal RCA. She undergoes successful coronary intervention to her proximal LAD and has an uncomplicated recovery from her infarct. Her echocardiogram demonstrates akinesia of the apex, but an overall EF estimated at 35–40%. She is established on dual anti-platelet therapy, ramipril, bisoprolol, and a statin.**

    What other therapy should she have?

    A. Spironalactone
    B. Epleronone
    C. ICD insertion
    D. CRT insertion
    E. PCI to her RCA

19. **A 45-year-old patient with a known diagnosis of AL amyloid presents to cardiology outpatient clinic. He is under the haematologists receiving chemotherapy for myeloma.**

    Which one of the following statements is true when there is cardiac involvement with amyloid?

    A. ACE inhibitor therapy is the cornerstone of treatment with cardiac involvement

    B. In endstage disease, cardiac transplantation in AL amyloid is relatively contraindicated

    C. Beta-blockers are used routinely

    D. With adjunctive chemotherapy, the prognosis for AL amyloid is good

    E. Diuretics should not be used because of profound hypotension

20. **A 50-year-old man with sarcoidosis is referred to the outpatient clinic from the respiratory clinic.**

    Which one of the following features would suggest cardiac involvement?

    A First-degree heart block

    B Dilated cardiomyopathy

    C Echo features suggestive of ARVC

    D E/A reversal on mitral inflow Doppler with an elevated E/E' on tissue Doppler imaging

    E All of the above

21. **You are asked to review a 65-year-old man with known pulmonary fibrosis who has been admitted under the chest physicians with an infection. He is not responding to broad-spectrum antibiotic therapy. He is a lifelong smoker. His 12-lead ECG demonstrates first-degree AV block with complete RBBB and a normal QRS axis. His CXR is of poor quality but could be consistent with fluid overload. Echocardiography demonstrates thinning of the septum and apex with overall moderate impairment of systolic function.**

    Which one of the following investigations is least likely to help with the underlying diagnosis?

    A. Cardiac catheterization

    B. BNP

    C. Serum ACE

    D. High-resolution CT chest

    E. Exercise ECG

22. **A 60-year-old female patient with previous lymphoma has been referred to cardiology clinic with breathlessness. She has previously received mediastinal radiotherapy.**

    Which one of the following is unlikely to be a cardiac cause of her symptoms?

    A. Constrictive pericarditis
    B. Aortic regurgitation
    C. Severe left main stem stenosis
    D. Complete heart block
    E. Pulmonary regurgitation

23. **A 52-year-old patient presents with breathlessness. He has had hypertension for many years but has been non-compliant with his medication. His echocardiogram demonstrates an EF of 70%, with marked concentric hypertrophy.**

    Which one of the following therapies is not appropriate?

    A. Ramipril
    B. Atenolol
    C. Irbesartan
    D. Amlodipine
    E. Bendroflumathiazide

24. **A 42-year-old Caucasian woman presents to the outpatient clinic when she is 10 weeks pregnant. This is her second pregnancy and was unplanned. Her first pregnancy was complicated by peripartum cardiomyopathy with moderate impairment of left ventricular systolic function. However, she did have complete resolution of systolic function 6 months after the birth of her first child.**

    Which one of the following statements is true?

    A. Her risk of death during this pregnancy is significantly increased
    B. Her risk of developing heart failure during the pregnancy is around 20%
    C. If she develops cardiomyopathy during this pregnancy, the likelihood of resolution of LV function after pregnancy is high
    D. Prophylactic use of ACE inhibitors is mandatory
    E. Early detection of heart failure by clinical examination during the pregnancy will be sufficiently sensitive to detect deteriorating LV function

1. B. A mineralocorticoid receptor antagonist (MRA) (spironolactone or epleronone) is the next choice of medication in patients with chronic symptomatic systolic heart failure (NYHA functional class II–IV) established on optimal ACE inhibitor and beta-blocker (BB). An angiotensin receptor blocker (ARB) is an alternative if an MRA is not tolerated. No indication for furosemide as the patient is not fluid overloaded.

2. E. The patient has severe AS; therefore an ACE inhibitor is contraindicated. Symptoms are probably due to AS and therefore further investigation is needed to assess for AVR. Angina symptoms should be treated with a BB in the interim. CRT-D is not indicated as severe AS needs addressing and EF is not less than 35% (NICE Guidelines).

3. D. The patient is not on optimal dosage of BB with a heart rate of 80 bpm; therefore titrate BB in the first instance before adding further agents. The target dose of bisoprolol is 10 mg or as close as tolerated. An MRA would be next line if the patient remains in NYHA class II+, followed by ivabradine if the heart rate remains >70 bpm.

4. B. The echocardiogram is suggestive of ischaemic heart disease being the aetiology of his symptoms. Angiography is the investigation of choice.

5. C. This is difficult as the 2012 ESC Guidelines and NICE Guidelines differ. The patient remains in NYHA class II despite optimal medication and an ECG shows sinus rhythm and LBBB. The ESC recommends CRT-D in patients in sinus rhythm with a QRS duration of ≥130 ms, LBBB QRS morphology, and an EF ≤30%. If she was in NYHA class III (or class IV with reasonable functionality), then CRT-P/D (defibrillators may be less desirable in advanced HF) is recommended for patients with a QRS ≥120 ms (LBBB) and an EF ≤35%, who are expected to survive with good functional status for >1 year. The ESC does not recommend dyssynchrony echo assessment.

Currently NICE recommends CRT for more advanced heart failure (NHYA class III–IV) with EF <35%, and distinguishes the need for a defibrillator based on cardiomyopathy of ischaemic origin. A QRS duration of 120–150 ms requires dyssynchrony on echo.

The patient's age is against transplant.

6. E. This patient has triple vessel disease with objective evidence of ischaemia. This is an indication for CABG. The ESC Guidelines recommend concomitant MVR if the patient has severe MR and LVEF >30% when planned for CABG.

7. D. ESC Guidelines suggest that if creatinine is 265–310 µmol/L or K^+ >5.5 mmol/L the dose of ACE inhibitor should be halved and blood chemistry should be monitored closely.

8. C. Transplant candidate if endstage heart disease with a life expectancy of 12–18 months, NYHA class III or IV heart failure, refractory to medical therapy including cardiac resynchronization therapy.

9. A. An ACE inhibitor should only be used in patients with adequate renal function (creatinine ≤221 mmol/L or ≤2.5 mg/dL or eGFR ≥30 mL/min/1.73 m^2) and a normal serum potassium level. Candesartan and epleronone are also contraindicated in view of the renal function. Furosemide is not indicated because of fluid status. Ivabradine requires an EF <35%.

H-ISDN is an alternative to ACE inhibitor/ARB when they are not tolerated, or can be considered in patients on maximal therapy and residual NYHA class II–IV symptoms and EF ≥35%.

10. C. The patient most likely has coronary vasculopathy. The incidence of this is 30–40% at 5 years. It progresses slowly, but as the heart is denervated a high clinical suspicion is required.

11. D. ACE is produced by vascular endothelial cells in the pulmonary vasculature (and systemic vascular endothelium). It converts angiotensin I to the active angiotensin II and promotes the production of bradykinin. An ACE inhibitor blocks the formation of angiotensin II and provides survival benefit in patients with LV systolic dysfunction. Angiotensin II stimulates the production of aldosterone and norepinephrine.

12. D. The mid-cavity anterior septum and anterior wall, as well as the entire apex, are thinned and akinetic in keeping with a regional wall motion abnormality in the LAD territory. There is severe LV systolic dysfunction.

13. C. TTE suggests moderate aortic stenosis, not severe AS, which is not a contraindication to starting an ACE inhibitor. All other answers are contraindications to starting an ACE inhibitor.

14. E. Septal ablation should be considered for relieving outflow tract obstruction with hypertrophic cardiomyopathy in patients with marked breathlessness (NYHA class III or IV) refractory to medical therapy. Although a change in medical therapy may help (e.g. addition of disopyramide), patients with a peak resting or exercise-induced gradient ≥50 mmHg should be referred to a specialist centre. Although there is some data to support the use of dual-chamber pacing, the overall consensus is that this should only be considered in certain subgroups, e.g. elderly patients or those at high operative risk. ICD implantation is used only to reduce the risk of sudden cardiac death in high-risk patients.

15. C. Young patients with no symptoms and no risk factors for sudden cardiac death do not require medical therapy. They should however be risk stratified with annual exercise testing to look for evidence of exercise induced arrhythmia (VT or AF) and a <20mmHg rise in blood pressure. Annual 24 hour Holter monitoring should also be performed to look for VT (>3 beats at a rate of >120bpm) or AF. AF is more common in the HCM population and should be treated medically (beta-blockers, verapamil or Amiodarone) and formal anticoagulation. Pregnancy is safe in patients without symptoms and usually culminates in a normal vaginal delivery. However, care should be delivered in a joint cardiac obstetric clinic. First degree relatives should be screened with ECG and echocardiography. Due to cases of late presentation of HCM, these tests should be repeated if normal.

16. A. Clinical features of right heart failure and a thickened left ventricle with evidence of restrictive filling (reversed E/A ratio and raised E/E') is suggestive of a restrictive cardiomyopathy. The presence of conduction disease and small QRS complexes in the context of echocardiographic evidence of left ventricular hypertrophy suggests amyloid deposition. Although demonstrating a plasma cell dyscrasia increases the likelihood of AL amyloid, the presence of cardiac amyloid can be demonstrated by endomyocardial biopsy. Myocardial perfusion imaging only demonstrates the presence of coronary artery disease. A left and right heart catheter can show restrictive physiology but not its aetiology.

17. D. The likely diagnosis is that of alcohol-related cardiomyopathy with by-stander coronary artery disease. Triple medical therapy with ACE inhibitors, beta-blockers and spironolactone has symptomatic and prognostic benefit and should be established early with appropriate dose uptitration. Although recovery of systolic function is seen with alcohol abstinence, medical therapy should be established together with abstinence advice. The indication for device therapy should be made once medical therapy is established and a reassessment of the patient's symptoms and left ventricular function is made. There is no strong data to support the use of formal anticoagulation in patients in sinus rhythm with dilated cardiomyopathy. The risk of concurrent alcohol use significantly reduces any benefits.

18. B. Epleronone is indicated post infarction with an ejection fraction of less than or equal to 40%. Spironalactone is used in patients with severe impairment of left ventricular systolic impairment (<35%) with NYHA class III symptoms. An ICD is not indicated for secondary prevention in the context of an acute infarct and where the ejection fraction is >35%. CRT is indicated only in symptomatic patients with a broad QRS (>150 ms) and echo features of dyssynchrony (if QRS is 120–150 ms). Coronary intervention on the RCA would only be indicated if the patient had angina symptoms and/or there was objective evidence of ischaemia.

19. B. Diuretics are the mainstay of treatment for cardiac failure and fluid overload in cardiac amyloid. ACE inhibitors are used, but with caution because of hypotension. Beta-blockers are used with caution because of the frequency of conduction disease. The prognosis of AL amyloid remains very poor despite treatment of the underlying haematological disorder with chemotherapy. Cardiac transplantation is complex in these patients and is associated with poor outcomes.

20. E. Cardiac sarcoid is a great mimic and can have a number of presentations. Conduction disease is common, as is sustained ventricular arrhythmia. The ventricular phenotype can be dilated or hypertrophic, as well as demonstrating regional wall motion abnormality and variability in ventricular wall thickness. Pericardial effusions, constriction, and valve disease have all been recognized.

21. E. Exercise ECG is likely to be non-diagnostic and insensitive for underlying coronary artery disease in view of baseline changes; a cardiac catheter will be diagnostic for an ischaemic aetiology. An elevated BNP would suggest a cardiac component to the acute presentation. Serum ACE and high-resolution CT of the chest looking for sarcoid could provide a unifying diagnosis. Sarcoid should be considered in patients with chronic lung disease and conduction disease on ECG.

22. E. Left-sided valve lesions are much more common than pulmonary or tricuspid valve involvement in post-radiotherapy patients. The reasons for this are unclear. Coronary disease is a risk due to intimal proliferation and accelerated atherosclerosis, even in the absence of traditional risk factors. Sick sinus syndrome and even complete heart block due to fibrosis have been seen. Constrictive pericarditis is a long-term sequela of radiation therapy and presents with signs of right heart failure. The treatment is pericardectomy.

23. B. The treatment for patients with hypertensive heart disease is adequate blood pressure control. However, not all agents are effective. ACE inhibitors and ARBs are the most effective, with calcium antagonists able to reduce LV mass. Atenolol is associated with a higher mortality because of its inability to prevent ventricular fibrillation.

24. B. Patients with previous peripartum cardiomyopathy with complete resolution of LV function have a low mortality risk in subsequent pregnancies. The risk of re-developing the cardiomyopathy is higher, with 20% presenting with heart failure with a reduction in the likelihood of resolution of LV function. ACE inhibitors are contraindicated in the first trimester of pregnancy. Examination findings in preganancy can be very misleading as systolic murmurs, third heart sound, and ankle oedema can be detected in normal pregnancy.

1. You are reviewing a 27-year-old male in clinic for the first time. On a routine health check 12 months previously he was found to have a restrictive perimembranous **VSD** on his echocardiogram. The jet velocity was measured at 5 m/s. There was no evidence of left ventricular dilatation and pulmonary pressures are not raised. He is asymptomatic. The rest of his echocardiogram confirmed a structurally normal heart apart from mild aortic regurgitation. You repeat the echocardiogram in clinic and there has been no change.

   What is the most appropriate follow-up?

   A. Advise him that this is an incidental finding which should not cause any problems and discharge him from clinic
   B. Advise that there is an increased risk of endocarditis but based on the current guidance there is no role for antibiotic prophylaxis and discharge him from clinic
   C. Arrange for follow-up with echocardiography in 12 months
   D. Advise him that although there are no problems at the moment it is advisable to close the VSD to reduce the risk of progressive haemodynamic change and risk of endocarditis. This can usually be done transcatheter
   E. Advise him that although there are no problems at the moment it is advisable to close the VSD to reduce the risk of progressive haemodynamic change and risk of endocarditis. This is usually done surgically

2. You are asked to review and explain the terminology on an echocardiogram report for a patient who has just returned to the ward having been admitted with stable but symptomatic **AV block**. The report states that there is **A–V and V–A discordance**.

   What is the underlying diagnosis?

   A. Congenitally corrected transposition of the great arteries (ccTGA)
   B. Transposition of the great arteries
   C. An atrioventricular defect with lack of AV valve offset
   D. Truncus arteriosus
   E. None of the above—the term describes a characteristic m-mode pattern of the AV valves in complete heart block

3. You are asked to review a **GUCH** patient at **03:00** who has
    directly attended the **ED** with palpitations and breathlessness.
    On his arrival, the notes are available and document a diagnosis
    of tricuspid atresia with Fontan surgery. The patient appears
    anxious but well and tells you the symptoms started 8 hours
    previously whilst he was eating. He is well perfused with heart
    rate 130 bpm, BP 110/70 mmHg, and saturations of 97% on room
    air. There are no clinical signs of heart failure. The ECG is shown
    in Figure 5.1. The QRS morphology is consistent with baseline
    ECGs. The patient is on warfarin with an INR of 2.7.

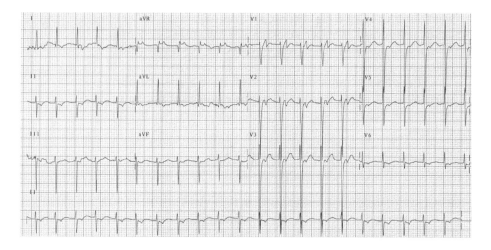

Figure 5.1

What is your management strategy?

A. Support with O_2 and IV fluids; look for underlying causes of tachycardia and especially
    sepsis; move to CCU and keep under close observation until morning

B. Give an adenosine bolus to diagnose the tachycardia; if an arrhythmia is proven, treat with
    oral beta-blocker and look for underlying causes

C. Give an adenosine bolus to diagnose the tachycardia; if an arrhythmia is proven, treat with
    intravenous amiodarone and look for underlying causes

D. It is likely that this represents a sinus tachycardia; reassure the patient; if routine bloods
    and CXR are normal, he can be discharged in the morning

E. This patient requires prompt DC cardioversion; adenosine can be attempted and IV fluids
    supplemented whilst making arrangements

4. You receive a letter from a **GP** asking if a patient requires
    follow-up in clinic. She is 35 years old and has not been seen
    since discharge from the paediatric cardiology services. She
    had a coarctation repair in childhood with no associated lesions.
    You have the surgical information, which documents a **Dacron**
    patch aortoplasty technique with excellent result and no residual
    stenosis. She is otherwise well with **BP 120/80 mmHg.** She has
    normal peripheral pulses and no murmurs. She has had two
    successful pregnancies.

    What should you advise the GP?

    A. She should have an echocardiogram and if this demonstrates normal structure and
        velocities in the descending aorta, based on normal blood pressure and clinical examination
        she does not require regular follow-up
    B. She does not require follow-up but should be referred to the pregnancy clinic if she
        decides to have more children
    C. She does not require any follow-up as surgical repair of coarctation has excellent long-term
        results
    D. She will require long-term follow-up in a specialist clinic; an MRI will be the investigation of
        choice to document the previous repair and any associated problems
    E. She should have an ambulatory blood pressure recording and if there is no evidence
        of hypertension there is no indication to explore any further; if there is evidence of
        hypertension she should have a CT scan to look for re-coarctation

5. A 33-year-old male has been admitted under the stroke physicians
    with an episode of transient left upper limb weakness, which
    lasted 1 hour after exercising at the gym. He has no prior medical
    history. He is a lifelong non-smoker with no important family
    history. He is very fit and plays competitive basketball. Blood
    tests reveal total cholesterol of 4.3 mmol/L. BP is 110/70 mmHg
    and ECG shows sinus rhythm with normal morphology. The
    stroke physicians arrange a CT head and echocardiogram. The
    CT head returns normal. You are asked to comment on the
    echocardiogram report which documents a structurally normal
    heart with no thrombus in the LA. The only finding is of an
    'aneurysmal' intra-atrial septum.

    What should you advise the stroke team?

    A. The patient should have a TOE as transthoracic echocardiography cannot rule out a
        cardiac source of thrombus
    B. Aneurysmal intra-atrial septum is a common and benign finding in young adults and the rest
        of the echocardiogram is reassuring. No further cardiac investigations are required
    C. They should arrange a Holter monitor to exclude a paroxysmal atrial arrhythmia which
        may have precipitated thrombus
    D. A bubble contrast echocardiogram would be the next investigation of choice
    E. Aneurysmal intra-atrial septums are associated with connective tissue disorders and he
        should have a CT aorta including neck vessels

6. **Which one of the following statements regarding the Fontan operation is correct?**

   A. It is a palliative procedure in patients with congenital cyanotic heart disease when a biventricular repair is not possible; the result is univentricular physiology with diversion of systemic venous return to the pulmonary arteries

   B. Patients should have a near-normal life expectancy as chronic cyanosis is corrected and the pulmonary vasculature is protected from systemic pressures

   C. It is one potential solution for transposition of the great arteries; systemic venous blood is diverted to the subpulmonary ventricle via an atrial baffle and pulmonary venous return is redirected to the systemic ventricle

   D. It is a corrective procedure for patients with functionally univentricular cyanotic heart disease; the end result is a biventricular repair

   E. It is a palliative procedure in patients with congenital cyanotic heart disease when a biventricular repair is not possible; the result is univentricular physiology with a systemic arterial to pulmonary shunt to increase pulmonary blood flow

7. **You are asked to review a 27-year-old female with complex congenital heart disease. She is normally managed at another centre, and limited information is available. She has had a number of operations in early life but has recently been well. Her parents tell you that she has 'one main pumping chamber'. The history is of deterioration over the last week with fevers and headache.**

   On examination the patient is cyanosed (baseline saturations 85% on room air) and agitated with GCS 13–15. Temperature is 38.4°C, BP is 120/80 mmHg, and heart rate is 100 bpm (regular). A bedside echocardiogram is attempted but the image quality is very poor. The ED team have initiated supportive treatment with high-flow O_2 and IV fluids. Blood cultures have been taken. The chest X-ray is suspicious for right basal consolidation.

   What would you advise?

   A. There is evidence of severe sepsis with compromise; in view of the complex congenital heart disease there is a risk of rapid decompensation and the patient should be moved to the ITU with a view to intubation if the hypoxia deteriorates

   B. The patient requires an immediate TOE as she is in a high-risk category for concomitant endocarditis and TTE is non-diagnostic

   C. In view of the temperature and reduced GCS she should have an urgent CT head

   D. After adequate blood cultures have been taken, initiate empirical antibiotics for pneumonia and move to CCU for supportive treatment; involve the ITU team in case of deterioration; aim for saturations >93% and plan for TOE when stabilized to rule out endocarditis

   E. Urgently contact the team she is under to establish the underlying diagnosis; aim for transfer if stabilized with supportive treatment

8. **When describing cardiac anatomy, what does the term 'situs solitus' refer to?**
   A. Normal orientation of the cardiac apex within the thorax, e.g. leftward pointing cardiac apex
   B. Normal orientation of the cardiac atria, e.g. morphological left atrium on the left and morphological right atrium on the right
   C. Mirror image of the cardiac structures and abdominal viscera, e.g. left-sided structures on the right and vice versa
   D. Normal orientation of the cardiac structures but with mirror images of the abdominal viscera
   E. Both atria are morphologically left-sided with associated cardiac and visceral organ abnormalities

9. **You are asked to review a 22-year-old male who has presented to the ED with sudden-onset chest pain and breathlessness. He has been diagnosed with a probable acute pulmonary embolism by the emergency team. They have asked for an echocardiogram to look for 'right heart strain' as he appears to be mildly compromised and they are considering thrombolysis if he decompensates. Auscultation of the heart sounds has revealed a loud continuous murmur and the CXR shows some pulmonary congestion.**

   What are you likely to see on echocardiography?
   A. A dilated and hyperdynamic RV with evidence of acute TR secondary to raised pulmonary pressure
   B. A jet of colour flow extending back into the RVOT from the pulmonary artery in the short-axis parasternal view
   C. A jet of colour extending from the right coronary sinus into the right ventricle
   D. A jet of colour across the apical interventircular septum in the four-chamber view
   E. A flail mitral valve leaflet with severe mitral regurgitation

10. **A haematology SHO contacts you regarding a patient with congenital cyanotic heart disease. The patient has trisomy 21 and an unrepaired complete AVSD with Eisenmenger physiology and chronic cyanosis. The patient was seen recently in clinic and was doing reasonably well. The full blood count has been highlighted to the haematology team as the patient has a haemoglobin (Hb) of 27. The haematology records document a previous venesection when the Hb was around the same figure and the patient had developed headaches thought to be due to hyperviscosity. The SHO would like some advice on whether they should arrange for daycase venesection to reduce the risk of hyperviscosity complications and symptoms.**

    What advice should you give?

    A. As the patient is asymptomatic there is no indication for venesection

    B. Daycase venesection should be arranged with volume replacement based on the Hb to prevent hyperviscosity complications

    C. The haematocrit (Hct) should be checked; if Hct > 65%, daycase isovolumic venesection is indicated

    D. The iron status should be checked first; in the presence of iron deficiency this should be treated first, prior to venesection

    E. The haematocrit and iron status should be checked: if Hct > 60% and the patient is iron replete, venesection should be performed: If the patient is iron deplete, venesection can be performed with pulsed iron and volume replacement

11. **You are approached by one of the adult congenital specialist nurses for advice regarding a patient with tetralogy of Fallot (ToF) who has contacted them directly. The patient, who is now 24 years old, had total surgical repair in childhood and has remained well since, but has recently been experiencing palpitations with associated presyncope. The symptoms are transient and there has been no syncope. There are no other relevant symptoms or reduction in exercise capacity. The echocardiogram from clinic a year previously showed moderate–severe PR and moderate RV dilatation. The nurse has performed an ECG which shows SR with first-degree AV block and RBBB (QRS 190 ms).**

    What is the most appropriate advice?

    A. The patient is at risk of malignant arrhythmias and sudden cardiac death; urgent haemodynamic assessment and consideration of an ICD is appropriate

    B. It is likely that the patient is experiencing paroxysmal SVTs or symptomatic ectopics; arrange an outpatient 24-hour tape

    C. It is common for patients with ToF repair to develop non-sustained RVOT arrhythmias at the site of the surgical scar, and beta-blockers are the initial treatment of choice for symptoms

    D. It is possible that the symptoms represent haemodynamic deterioration; an echocardiogram should be arranged to document progression of PR and RV dilatation

    E. High degrees of AV block/sinus node dysfunction are probably due to the scar from the VSD patch; the best investigation is an implantable loop recorder with a view to a permanent pacemaker

12. **One of the stroke physicians asks your advice regarding a 45-year-old man admitted with a stroke. The patient is overweight with known hypertension and raised lipids. He is a non-smoker. Carotid Doppler scans show no atheroma. The stroke physicians have performed a 24-hour tape which has shown clear runs of asymptomatic paroxysmal AF. They have also requested a bubble contrast echo which has demonstrated complete opacification of the left heart with Valsalva release. The heart is structurally normal apart from moderate LVH and a left atrial area of 30 cm^2. The patient is currently on antiplatelet therapy, but they are keen to know what the immediate strategy would be from the cardiac point of view.**

    A. There is a large PFO which represents a significant risk factor for recurrent stroke; once the patient has recovered, inpatient transcatheter PFO closure is indicated
    B. There is clear evidence of paroxysmal AF: in the context of stroke and cardiovascular risk factors, we would recommend anticoagulation once beyond the acute risk of haemorrhagic transformation; no further treatment for the PFO is required whilst on anticoagulation
    C. The patient is young and should have pulmonary vein isolation and a flutter ablation with transcatheter left atrial appendage closure and PFO closure
    D. TOE is the next step to confirm the presence and anatomy of the shunt
    E. Short episodes of AF can be seen in the context of an acute illness: the patient should have aggressive cardiovascular risk factor modification and BP control with ACE inhibitors; further ambulatory ECGs should be peformed when he has recovered as the AF may have been treated

13. **One of the medical students asks you what a Fontan operation consists of.**

    What is your answer?

    A. A palliative procedure when a biventricular surgical repair is not possible: the systemic venous blood is directly routed into the pulmonary arteries bypassing the ventricle
    B. When a biventricular surgical repair is not possible the systemic venous blood is directly routed into the pulmonary arteries bypassing the ventricle; life expectancy is near normal
    C. It is a procedure for the treatment of transposition of the great arteries but is no longer performed; the systemic venous blood is routed via baffles to the morphological left ventricle (subpulmonary ventricle) and the pulmonary venous blood is routed to the morphological RV (systemic ventricle)
    D. It consists of an SVC-to-PA shunt to increase pulmonary blood flow in congenital cyanotic heart disease when pulmonary flow is low
    E. It consists of a subclavian-to-PA shunt to increase pulmonary blood flow in congenital cyanotic heart disease when pulmonary flow is low

14. You are following up a 33-year-old male in clinic who was referred by the GP for increasing breathlessness and intermittent palpitations. A transthoracic echocardiogram was performed which revealed moderate right heart dilatation but no abnormality of the right-sided valves. Right ventricular systolic pressure was estimated at 30 mmHg. He has no respiratory problems and is a lifelong non-smoker. He is slim with good echocardiogram images, and careful interrogation of the intra-atrial and ventricular septum shows no evidence of a colour flow.

    What is a likely differential diagnosis?

    A. ASD
    B. VSD
    C. PFO
    D. Primary respiratory disease with right heart changes
    E. PDA

15. You are following up a 28-year-old male in clinic who was referred by his GP for increasing breathlessness and intermittent palpitations. He has come back for the result of his TOE which has shown evidence of a superior sinus venosus ASD with normal pulmonary venous drainage and moderate right heart dilatation. He asks you about the likely treatment.

    A. Transcatheter ASD device closure
    B. Surgical ASD closure
    C. ACE inhibitor treatment to reduce the shunt and protect the right heart
    D. Monitoring in clinic for signs of severe right heart dilatation
    E. Stenting of the SVC to commit blood into the RA

16. Which one of the following patients would you advise to avoid pregnancy?

    A. A 25-year-old with repaired ToF and severe pulmonary regurgitation with a mildly dilated and mildly impaired right ventricle
    B. A 32-year-old with idiopathic pulmonary arterial hypertension, which has responded well to bosentan, who has a right atrial to right ventricular pressure drop of 45 mmHg
    C. A 39-year-old patient with moderate mitral regurgitation and good left ventricular function
    D. An 18-year-old with a single-ventricle circulation and a total cavopulmonary connection operation for tricuspid atresia, normally saturated and with good LV function
    E. A 28-year-old with a Senning repair of the transposition of the great arteries with mildly reduced systemic ventricular function and mild to moderate tricuspid regurgitation

17. **A 36-year-old patient with repaired ToF wishes to become pregnant and asks you about the likelihood of her child being born with a congenital heart defect. She has no family history of congenital heart disease.**

    What is the approximate risk of her child having congenital heart disease?

    A. 1–2%

    B. 8–10%

    C. 50%

    D. 4–5%

    E. No more than the general population. Most cases are sporadic.

18. **A GP writes to you to ask which contraceptive is advisable for her 35-year-old patient with a mechanical mitral valve replacement. She has had one child and several miscarriages because of taking warfarin. She does not wish to become pregnant again.**

    What is the best method of contraception for this patient?

    A. Sterilization

    B. Condoms

    C. Mirena intra-uterine system

    D. Depo Provera

    E. Combined oral contraceptive pill

19. **In current regulations, which of the following drugs is absolutely contraindicated in pregnancy?**

    A. Atenolol

    B. Simvastatin

    C. Aspirin

    D. Amlodipine

    E. Clopidogrel

20. **A 35-year-old woman with a history of atrioventricular nodal tachycardia presents in premature labour at 36 weeks with a narrow complex tachycardia at 180 bpm (see Figure 5.2).**

    What is the most appropriate drug to use after vagal manoeuvres and adenosine?

    A. Esmolol

    B. Amiodarone

    C. Verapamil

    D. Digoxin

    E. Flecainide

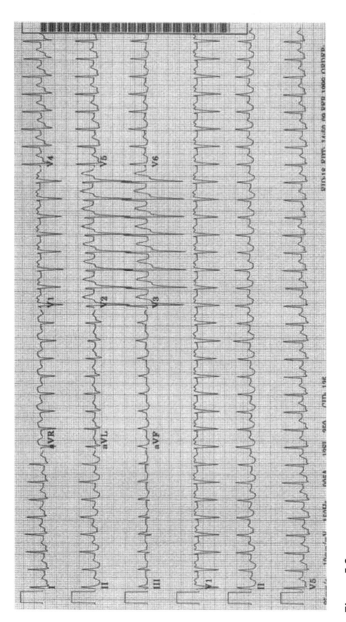

Figure 5.2

21. **Which of the following are the first-, second-, and third-line drugs to use in pregnancy-induced hypertension with no other problems?**

    A. Methyldopa, labetolol, nifedipine
    B. Nifedipine, captopril, bendroflumethazide
    C. Metoprolol, methyldopa, bendroflumethazide
    D. Enalapril, labetolol, doxazosin
    E. Enalapril, methyldopa, labetolol

22. **A 24-year-old woman who has a mechanical mitral valve replacement and requires warfarin 4 mg od comes to your clinic, seeking advice about becoming pregnant. She has heard that warfarin is dangerous in pregnancy.**

    What is the best anticoagulation regime in pregnancy to protect her from valve thrombosis?

    A. Warfarin throughout pregnancy switching to heparin 2–3 weeks before delivery
    B. Low molecular weight heparin for weeks 6–12 and warfarin for weeks 12–38, switching to heparin 2 weeks before delivery
    C. Low molecular weight heparin throughout with four-weekly monitoring of anti-Xa levels
    D. Low molecular weight heparin and aspirin throughout with four-weekly monitoring of anti-Xa levels
    E. Warfarin throughout pregnancy with switch to heparin once in labour

23. **A 28-year-old woman with Marfan syndrome presents 28 weeks pregnant, having been lost to follow-up, with a 47 mm sinus of Valsalva measurement on her echocardiogram (see Figure 5.3). There is a family history of aortic dissection.**

    Which one of the following would be the best recommended mode of delivery?

    A. Normal vaginal delivery with analgesia only as required because of the haemodynamic changes induced by epidural anaesthesia
    B. Normal vaginal delivery with surgeon on standby and a low threshold for epidural analgesia
    C. Vaginal delivery with elective combined spinal/epidural and completely passive second stage(pushing stage) with lift-out forceps/ventouse
    D. Vaginal delivery with elective combined spinal/epidural and up to 30 minutes of pushing
    E. Elective Caesarean section with cardiothoracic surgeon on standby

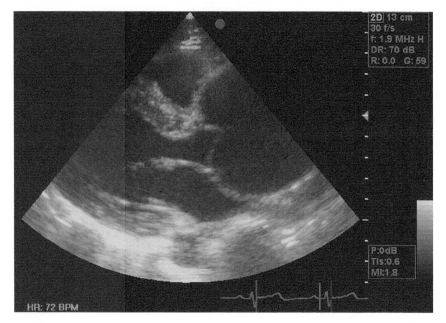

Figure 5.3

24. **A 25-year old woman who is 35 weeks pregnant is referred to
your clinic because of increasing shortness of breath, palpitations
on exertion, and a murmur. A soft non-radiating ejection systolic
murmur is heard loudest in expiration at the left sternal edge.
Pulse is 90 bpm and normal in character. Blood pressure in the
right arm is 104/62 mmHg. Non-pitting ankle oedema is present.
The ECG shows sinus rhythm with left axis deviation and Q
waves in lead III. The ST segments are quite flat inferolaterally
with widespread T-wave inversion. There are several premature
ventricular complexes. Echocardiography does not show the
aortic valve clearly, but peak velocity across the LV outflow tract
is 1.8m/s.**

    Which one of the following is the most appropriate next investigation?

    A. Modified Bruce treadmill testing to assess the significance of the likely mild aortic stenosis
    B. Nothing—all the above are normal findings in pregnancy and the patient should be
    reassured
    C. Cardiac magnetic resonance imaging—the patient may have a right ventricular
    cardiomyopathy
    D. Holter monitoring to look for arrhythmias
    E. Transoesophageal echo to look at the aortic valves in more detail

25. **A 42-year-old woman presents 38 weeks pregnant with her fourth child with a 1 hour history of severe sudden-onset dull central chest pain associated with sweating and dyspnoea. She is diabetic, obese, and a smoker. The ECG shows 4 mm of ST elevation in the anterior leads.**

    What is the ideal management?

    A. Urgent thrombolysis to avoid the radiation risk of coronary angiography to the baby
    B. Primary angioplasty optimally with a drug eluting stent
    C. Primary angioplasty optimally avoiding a drug eluting stent
    D. Emergency delivery and subsequent standard primary angioplasty
    E. Use morphine, nitrates, aspirin, and heparin, and try to avoid intervention and inducing labour

26. **A 30-year-old woman presents to the clinic 17 weeks pregnant and becoming increasingly breathless. The LVEDD is 6.1 cm and the EF is estimated at 25%.**

    Which one of the following statements is false?

    A. Termination of pregnancy is justified on medical grounds
    B. An ACE inhibitor and beta-blocker should be started as soon as possible
    C. Prescribing a nitrate and hydralazine may cause the symptoms to subside
    D. The patient should rest and be admitted to hospital for this if necessary
    E. Premature delivery is likely

27. **A 19-year-old woman was born with transposition of the great arteries and had a Mustard repair. She has been well throughout her pregnancy, but presents at 37 weeks with a week of worsening dull central chest pain on exertion, associated with shortness of breath.**

    Which one of the following statements is false?

    A. The woman is probably suffering from coronary insufficiency because the hypertrophied right ventricle only has a single-vessel blood supply
    B. This is an acute coronary syndrome in pregnancy, which may be a dissection; the patient should go to the catheterization laboratory
    C. The patient should be treated with bed rest and antianginals
    D. The patient should be induced if the cervix is favourable
    E. The baby should be delivered

28. You are called to the labour ward because a 34-year-old woman has become breathless and orthopnoeic 2 hours after delivery. She is pain free. On examination she is tachycardic, tachypnoeic, and has a gallop rhythm. Blood pressure is 136/86 mmHg. On auscultation of her chest she has fine inspiratory crackles to the mid-zones.

    What is the most likely diagnosis?

    A. Pulmonary embolism
    B. Amniotic fluid embolus
    C. Peripartum cardiomyopathy
    D. Myocardial infarction
    E. Tachyarrhythmia precipitating ventricular decompensation

29. A 27-year-old woman presents at 26 weeks gestation in pulmonary oedema. She recently moved to the UK from Pakistan but was previously well. An echocardiogram showed mitral valve disease. The MV area is 1.0 cm², mean gradient is 25 mmHg, and PHT is 220 ms.

    What is the most appropriate treatment?

    A. Deliver the baby by Caesarean section and arrange balloon mitral valvuloplasty
    B. Deliver the baby by Caesarean section and arrange mitral valve replacement
    C. Arrange urgent mitral valve replacement surgery
    D. Arrange an urgent balloon mitral valvuloplasty
    E. Bed rest, give diuretics, and treat with a beta-blocker

30. A 38-year-old woman presents 34 weeks pregnant to the ED in atrial fibrillation. Blood pressure is 110/62 mmHg. Echocardiograpy and blood test results are normal.

    Which of the following is not a good first line of action?

    A. IV amiodarone
    B. IV flecainide
    C. DC cardioversion
    D. IV labetolol
    E. IV digoxin

1. C. Restrictive VSDs, by definition, have no haemodynamic consequences. There is an increased risk of endocarditis but no role for prophylactic antibiotics based on current guidance. They can cause aortic valve prolapse (usually right coronary cusp) and progressive dysfunction as a result of the Venturi effect of the high-velocity jet and turbulence below the AV. Patients with evidence of any degree of AV regurgitation require close follow-up for progression as surgical repair of the VSD is indicated prior to irreversible valve damage.

2. A. The terms are based on the sequential segmental approach of describing anatomy based on the cardiac component and connections from atria to ventricles (A–V) and ventricles to great vessels (V–A).

A–V and V–A discordance describes ccTGA where the ventricles are inverted. If the RA connects to the morphological LV (through the 'mitral' valve) (see Figure 5.4) and the LA connects to the morphological RV (through the 'tricuspid' valve), this is A–V discordance. If the LV then connects to the PA and the RV connects to the aorta, this is V–A discordance.

AV block is common in patients with ccTGA and may be the presenting complaint in an undiagnosed adult. The other common presentation is heart failure, as the RV and TV are not designed for systemic work and eventually 'wear out'.

In TGA there is A–V concordance but V–A discordance.

3. E. Tachyarrhythmias in patients with Fontan circulation is a medical emergency. Although they can appear well, there is a risk of rapid decompensation. These patients depend on LA contraction and effective left-sided diastolic haemodynamics to maintain pulmonary flow. Dehydration and arrhythmia can be fatal and prompt return of sinus rhythm is paramount.

4. D. The Dacron patch aortoplasty technique has been shown to be associated with a risk of late aneurysm formation. Therefore there may not be any evidence of re-coarctation but a risk of aneurysm in this patient. MRI will be the best follow-up modality as it will provide structural and physiological data without radiation. The brain should also be scanned to look for berry aneurysms. If a patient has had a coarctation stent, MRI does not have the resolution of CT in detecting stent fracture and the latter may be preferable depending on the situation.

The other common surgical techniques for coarctation repair are end-to-end anastomosis and subclavian flap repair (left sublavian artery is used to augment coarctation site). These can be associated with re-coarctation or pseudo-aneurysm and require long-term follow-up for BP control and the possibility of transcatheter stenting.

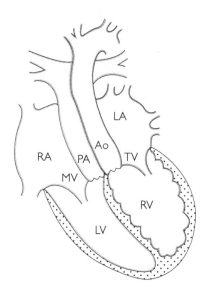

Figure 5.4 Isolated ccTGA: Ao, aorta; LA, left atrium; LV, left ventricle; PA, pulmonary artery; MV, mitral valve; RA, right atrium; RV, right ventricle; TV, tricuspid valve.

Reproduced from *The Oxford Specialist Handbook of Adult Congenital Heart Disease*, eds Sara Thorne and Paul Clift, © 2011 with permission of Oxford University Press.

5. D. The case describes a young patient without any risk factors for cardiovascular disease who clinically has had a TIA. In these patients a paradoxical embolus via a PFO should be considered. 'Aneurysmal' intra-atrial septum describes an excessively mobile septum (septal excursion ≥10 mm with a base diameter ≥15 mm on echo). Aneurysmal intra-atrial septums commonly have associated PFO or fenestrations, and so the possibility of a communication should be suspected if seen on echo. PFO with an aneurysmal septum confers a higher risk of stroke then PFO alone.

A well-performed bubble contrast echocardiogram (with sniff and Valsalva) is the investigation of choice to confirm the presence of a right-to-left shunt at atrial level.

6. A. The Fontan operation is a palliative procedure in patients with complex cyanotic heart disease when a biventricular reapir is not possible. These patients have univentricular physiology with mixing of pulmonary and systemic blood in a dominant ventricle (a rudimentary ventricle is often present connected via a 'VSD'). Life expectancy is not normal. The procedure consists of redirection of systemic venous blood to the pulmonary arteries (although there are a number of technical variations). The current modification is the total cavopulmonary connection (TCPC) (Figure 5.5).

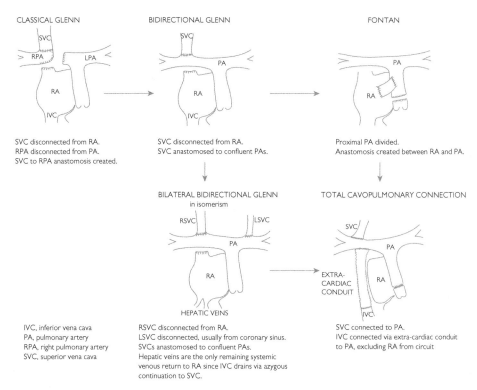

CLASSICAL GLENN

SVC disconnected from RA.
RPA disconnected from PA.
SVC to RPA anastomosis created.

BIDIRECTIONAL GLENN

SVC disconnected from RA.
SVC anastomosed to confluent PAs.

FONTAN

Proximal PA divided.
Anastomosis created between RA and PA.

BILATERAL BIDIRECTIONAL GLENN
in isomerism

TOTAL CAVOPULMONARY CONNECTION

IVC, inferior vena cava
PA, pulmonary artery
RPA, right pulmonary artery
SVC, superior vena cava

RSVC disconnected from RA.
LSVC disconnected, usually from coronary sinus.
SVCs anastomosed to confluent PAs.
Hepatic veins are the only remaining systemic
venous return to RA since IVC drains via azygous
continuation to SVC.

SVC connected to PA.
IVC connected via extra-cardiac conduit
to PA, excluding RA from circuit

Figure 5.5 Glenn and Fontan operations. TCPC is the modern modification.

Reproduced from *The Oxford Textbook of Medicine* (5th edn), eds David A. Warrell, Timothy M. Cox, John D. Firth, © 2010 with permission of Oxford University Press.

Surgery for TGA to redirect blood via baffles (atrial switch) is named either the Mustard procedure (prosthetic baffles) or the Senning procedure (intrinsic atrial tissue baffles). These approaches have been superseded by the more successful arterial switch procedure.

Systemic arterial-to-pulmonary shunts (e.g. Balock–Taussig shunt) can be used in a staged approach to palliate a patient until a Fontan procedure is completed.

7. C. This question emphasizes the risk of cerebral abscess in patients with cyanotic heart disease. Patients with cyanotic heart disease and evidence of sepsis with neurological deterioration require urgent investigation for cerebral abscess.

This patient has no evidence of significant haemodynamic compromise. Saturations of 85% may be normal for a patient with univentricular physiology (mixing of systemic and pulmonary blood) and balanced pulmonary and systemic circulations. Clearly it would be important to treat potential chest sepsis and rule out endocarditis.

8. B. Situs solitus refers to a normal orientation of the cardiac structure and abdominal viscera relative to the midline. For congenital heart disease the anatomy is defined from the atria (e.g. the morphological left atrium can be identified by its appendage but may be on the right side, this is situs inversus).

9. C. This case describes a young patient with sinus of Valsalva aneurysm rupture (acute symptoms, pulmonary congestion, and continuous murmur). Answer B describes a PDA which can be associated with a continuous murmur and endocarditis but not such an acute presentation. PE does not cause pulmonary congestion or a continuous murmur.

10. A. Polycythaemia is a physiological adaptive process to chronic cyanosis. Venesection should be avoided unless there are clear hyperviscosity symptoms. Venesection is not associated with a reduced risk of stroke and may cause iron deficiency and circulatory collapse without careful volume replacement.

11. A. The duration of the QRS is proportional to the size of the RV. It has been shown that a QRS >180 ms is a highly sensitive marker for VT and SCD in previous ToF repair (SCD accounts for a third of late deaths).

This patient's case should be urgently discussed and the option of an ICD considered. Haemodynamic assessment with echocardiography is also important as the PR or RV dilatation may have progressed, with the need for PV intervention.

Non-sustained VT is common but is not an indicator of SCD risk. Antiarrhythmics are not indicated if the patient is asymptomatic. The VT is normally of RVOT origin (infundibulectomy or VSD patch).

Development of major arrhythmias (AF/flutter and sustained VT) normally reflects haemodynamic deterioration (PR, RV dilatation) and therefore haemodynamic assessment and correction of the lesion can correct the arrhythmia (with the option of surgical/catheter ablation).

12. B. This case describes a relatively young patient with a number of risk factors for stroke. Despite having risk factors for atherosclerosis, because of his age (and clear carotid Doppler scans) other foci for embolic stroke have been pursued. Two possibilities have been identified: left atrial thrombus as a result of AF or a paradoxical embolus via the PFO. The question asks for the **immediate** strategy. Anticoagulation protects against both sources of embolus and so is the immediate treatment of choice. PFO closure will not protect against LA thrombus due to PAF and anticoagulation would still be required.

Complex ablation and device treatment may be a future option based on progress, but needs careful discussion.

TOE is not required after a suggestive positive bubble test, which is the preferred modality to confirm a PFO. Periprocedural TOE is used to guide transcatheter closure.

The AF is likely to be due to uncontrolled hypertension (LVH) and strict control with an ACE inhibitor can reduce the AF burden.

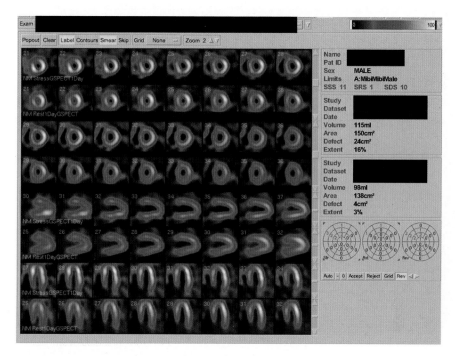

Plate 1 See also Fig. 7.11.

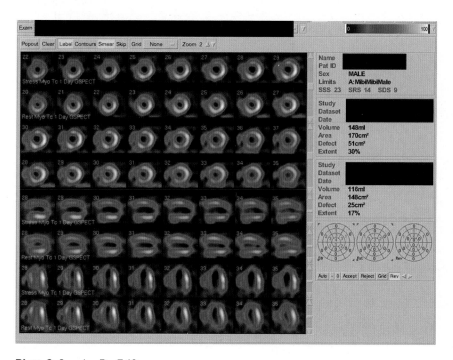

Plate 2 See also Fig. 7.12.

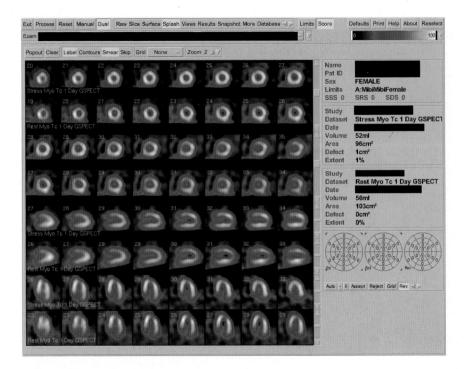

Plate 3 See also Fig. 7.13.

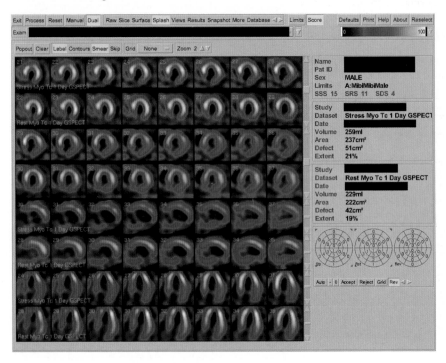

Plate 4 See also Fig. 7.14.

13. A.

- A describes the Fontan operation for complex congenital cyanotic heart disease when a biventricular repair is not possible. There are a number of modifications. The modern technique is the total cavopulmonary connection which routes blood directly to the PAs avoiding the atrium.
- B: the procedure is palliative, i.e. life expectancy is reduced.
- C describes an atrial switch (Senning or Mustard) operation for TGA.
- D describes a Glenn shunt. This can be part of a staged Fontan operation which would require IVC blood rerouting to the PA for completion (either via an extracardiac conduit or a lateral tunnel).
- E describes the Blalock–Tausigg shunt.

14. A.   Secundum and primum (AVSD) defects can be clearly seen on transthoracic echo. However, sinus venosus defects may not be seen. This patient has signs and a suspicion of an ASD physiology type left-to-right shunt. This includes anomalous pulmonary venous drainage, which is associated with superior sinus venosus ASD. He should have further imaging in the form of TOE or CT/CMR to identify the pulmonary venous drainage and look for a less obvious ASD.

PFOs cause no haemodynamic anatomical change. Haemodynamically significant VSDs result in left ventricular volume loading and increased pulmonary flow with eventual pulmonary hypertension, as do PDAs (not right-sided volume loading).

15. B.   This patient has a sinus venosus ASD with symptoms and evidence of haemodynamic anatomical change. The defect is in the superior atrium at the entrance of the SVC into the RA (almost as if the SVC overrides the atrial septum).

Currently, transcatheter solutions are not available and surgery is the treatment of choice. Sinus venosus ASDs are often associated with anomalous pulmonary venous drainage which requires surgical correction.

If the shunt is not corrected, this may result in irreversible right heart dysfunction, pulmonary hypertension (late), or the development of atrial arrhythmias such as AF which complicate the situation.

ACE inhibitors reduce LA pressure, and therefore in theory can reduce the shunt, but this is not a suitable treatment.

16. B.   Pregnancy is well tolerated in most patient groups, even those with a Fontan circulation. It is extremely high risk in patients with severe systemic ventricular impairment, those with a dilated aorta, those with pulmonary hypertension, and those with severe obstructive valve lesions due to the high risk of maternal morbidity. These patients should be counselled against pregnancy. The risk of mortality in patients with pulmonary hypertension is high. It has remained one of the leading causes of death in pregnancy for many decades, along with myocardial infarction, aortic dissection, and peripartum cardiomyopathy. Furthermore, bosentan is contraindicated in pregnancy.

17. D.   Most congenital heart disease is multifactorial in origin. There are some familial syndromes and some with autosomal dominant inheritance but generally the risk of inheritance of many lesions is 4–5%. Patients with left-sided obstructive lesions and atrioventricular septal defects have a slightly higher risk of passing on a defect—in the region of 6–8%. The risk of defects being passed on by fathers is lower.

18. C. Patients with heart disease are often unaware of the most suitable contraception for them and the quality of advice offered is universally poor. Generally speaking, progesterones (including the morning-after pill) are safe for all cardiac conditions. Condoms have a high failure rate and should not be used in women in whom avoiding pregnancy is important. The combined pill should be avoided in those in whom clotting is hazardous, i.e. dilated cardiomyopathy, Fontan, Mustard/Senning, AF/atrial flutter, previous clot, cyanosis/shunt, pulmonary hypertension, and mechanical valves. The progesterone implant and progesterone coil (Mirena IUS) are well tolerated and much more effective than sterilization. Consideration needs to be given to women on warfarin because of the risk of heavy/irregular bleeding with the mini-pill or Depo. Additionally Depo and implanted devices can result in painful bruising at the site of injection. The Mirena coil results in a lighter period, which is useful for women on warfarin and is highly effective.

19. B. Statins are categorized by the FDA as Category X because they inhibit mevalonic acid and have been shown to cause skeletal abnormalities in fetuses as well as resulting in fetal death. Although it has been proposed that statins in pregnancy may have benefits for treatment of pre-eclampsia this remains unproven and is not an accepted clinical indication. Atenolol, clopidogrel, and amlodipine can be used in pregnancy if the benefit to the mother outweighs the risk to the fetus. Aspirin is best avoided in the first trimester but is safe later in pregnancy in doses of <150 mg od.

20. A. Tachyarrhythmias in labour are often catecholamine driven and therefore beta-blockers are the most effective and appropriate drugs. The short half-life of esmolol is useful as it terminates the tachyarrhythmia without having a prolonged effect on labour. The others are less likely to be effective. Amiodarone is contraindicated in pregnancy.

21. A. No drugs have been subjected to randomized controlled trials in pregnant women so safety data are based on observational data in humans and animal fetuses. FDA categorization is helpful. Briefly, Category A drugs are proven to be safe in clinical trials; no drugs are in this category. Category B drugs are those in which there has been no evidence of harm from animal or human observational studies. Category C drugs are those in which abnormalities have been shown in animals given the drug but not seen in humans. Category D indicates evidence of risk to human fetuses, but benefit to the mother may still outweigh risk to the fetus. Category X drugs are harmful to the human fetus and benefit to the mother does not outweigh risk to the fetus. Methyldopa (Category B) is safe in pregnancy and is the first-line drug used for hypertension. Beta-blockers (Categories B and C) can cause intra-uterine growth retardation and neonatal hypoglycaemia, but are frequently used with four-weekly growth scans. Nifedipine (Category C) has not been shown to cause problems in humans. ACE inhibitors (category D) are teratogenic and later cause renal abnormalities, oligohydramnios, and limb contractures. Thiazides are not safe in pregnancy as they result in neonatal thrombocytopenia, jaundice, hyponatraemia, and bradycardia. Doxazosin is Category C but is not often used as there are other alternatives.

22. A. Warfarin crosses the placenta and can cause spontaneous abortion, stillbirth, neonatal death, and prematurity. In addition, warfarin is teratogenic, particularly in weeks 6–9, resulting in warfarin embryopathy (nasal hypoplasia, saddle-shaped nasal bridge, skeletal defects, short fingers and toes, low birth weight, and developmental delay). However, the incidence of embryopathy in fetuses where the mother has been given warfarin in doses <5 mg daily is zero. Therefore the risk for this particular patient, who is on 4 mg of warfarin, is low. Heparin does not cross the placenta and so is safe for the fetus, but there is an increased incidence of valve thrombosis which can result in death. Low molecular weight heparin has not been shown to avoid this problem, although the incidence of valve thrombosis is lower.

The position of the valve should also be considered. The mitral valve is more likely to thrombose than the aortic valve, and pregnancy is a hypercoagulable state with increased activation of prothrombin 1 and 2, TAT (thrombin–antithrombin complex), and D-dimer. Therefore the safest option for this patient is to continue warfarin throughout pregnancy. Warfarin should be stopped several weeks before delivery to reduce the risk of neonatal intracranial haemorrhage. Warfarin takes several weeks to be metabolized by the fetal liver.

23. E. The risk of dissection in pregnant Marfan patients is high (approximately 10% with sinus of Valsalva measuring >40 mm, compared with 1% if <40 mm). All patients should be on beta-blockers throughout pregnancy. Aortic dissection is one of the four major causes of death in pregnancy (which is rare) and can occur in women with normal aortas. Hormonal changes result in histological changes in the aorta and an increased risk of dissection. A patient with a family history of dissection has an additional high risk of dissection. Even though Caesarean section results in greater haemodynamic shifts than vaginal birth, the safest mode of delivery in this case would be to perform a Caesarean section in controlled circumstances with cardiothoracic standby in case aortic surgery is required as an emergency. Patients with significant aortopathy associated with other conditions, such as a bicuspid aortic valve, should also be treated with caution. Epidural anaesthesia results in hypotension, but if it is done by a careful titration technique with IV fluids and invasive monitoring by an experienced anaesthetist this can be overcome. In this case a combined spinal/epidural using the technique described would be recommended.

24. B. History and examination can be misleading as dyspnoea, palpitations, and peripheral oedema are common in pregnant women and hypotension and a collapsing pulse are the norm. Over >90% of pregnant women will have an ejection systolic murmur. Sinus tachycardia, right bundle branch block, and premature ventricular and atrial complexes are common in pregnancy, and in the third trimester the ECG often shows left axis deviation, Q III, T III, and inferolateral ST depression, and T-wave inversion. Velocities across the outflow tract in pregnancy are usually increased because of the increased volume load, and chamber sizes on the echocardiogram are increased.

25. C. Myocardial infarction in pregnancy is rare but is increasing because mothers are tending to be older with increased incidences of obesity, diabetes, and smoking. Coronary dissection can occur, but now myocardial infarction due to coronary atheroma is more common. The adverse haemodynamics in pregnancy plus increased oxygen consumption and hypercoagulability increase the risk. Mortality is high (around 11%, although it is now decreasing in the primary PCI era). The aim should be to save the mother's life and so radiation is not a concern. The life of the baby depends on survival of the mother (fetal mortality is approximately 9%, mostly due to maternal death). Conservative management is not appropriate. Interventional strategies and the subsequent need for antiplatelet agents are complicated and depend on a number of factors. The need for Clopidogrel precludes regional anaesthesia which is desirable post infarct. The Genous stent would currently require the shortest duration of dual antiplatelet treatment for around a week compared to 28 days for a bare metal stent.

26. B. ACE inhibitors are absolutely contraindicated in the second and third trimesters of pregnancy because of the risk of renal defects, oligohydramnios, and limb contractures.

Hydralazine and nitrate is a safe alternative. Rest (bed rest in hospital) is likely to be required in this case. The aim would be for the fetus to reach viability without compromising the mother. Termination of pregnancy would be justified in this case as there is a high risk of pulmonary oedema, intractable heart failure, stroke, and fetal loss. Patients with occult left ventricular dysfunction and obstructive valve disease usually present around this point in gestation as this is when their increase in cardiac output and plasma volume during pregnancy begins to peak (apart from in labour). The haemodynamic changes in pregnancy are profound. Hormonally mediated increases in blood volume, red cell mass, and heart rate result in a significant increase in cardiac output. Cardiac output peaks during the second trimester, and then remains constant until term. Circulating prostaglandins and other gestational hormones, and the low-resistance vascular bed of the placenta, result in decreases in peripheral vascular resistance and blood pressure. Blood pressure reaches its nadir in the middle of the second trimester and then begins to rise again towards term.

27. B.   Congenital heart disease affects 0.8% of live births and 85% of patients now survive to adulthood. Approximately 70% patients seen in cardiac antenatal clinics are those with congenital heart disease.

Patients with atrial switch repair of transposition of the great arteries have a single right ventricle, which does not cope well with the demands of pregnancy. Coronary insufficiency can occur because of a mismatch between myocardial oxygen supply and demand. Short-term conservative treatment is acceptable but delivery should be expedited if possible, and certainly at 37 weeks gestation.

28. C.   This is a typical picture of peripartum cardiomyopathy (often undiagnosed dilated cardiomyopathy, which decompensates at this time of extreme increase in preload). The largest haemodynamic changes in pregnancy occur in the post-partum period. During labour and delivery, pain and uterine contractions result in additional increases in cardiac output and blood pressure. Immediately after delivery, relief of caval compression and autotransfusion from the emptied and contracted uterus produce a further increase in cardiac output (50–70% more than baseline overall). Most haemodynamic changes of pregnancy resolve by 2 weeks post-partum.

Myocardial infarction in pregnancy is generally accompanied by pain, and pulmonary embolus does not result in signs of left heart failure. Tachyarrhythmia in pregnancy is common and is not usually associated with ventricular decompensation. Amniotic fluid embolus is rare and presents with shortness of breath leading to hypotension, cyanosis, and cardiac arrest.

29. D.   If the patient is already in pulmonary oedema this will continue to worsen through pregnancy, so diuretics etc. will only be a temporary relief. The outcome for a fetus delivered at 26 weeks is poor and therefore delivery is not desirable at this gestation. The treatment of choice is balloon mitral valvuloplasty by a skilled operator. Balloon mitral valvuloplasty is highly effective in pregnancy and safe. If there is severe mitral regurgitation at the end of the procedure this will be much better tolerated in progressing pregnancy than severe mitral stenosis. Note that the increased preload of pregnancy needs to be taken into account when assessing mitral stenosis. Peak and mean gradients will be extremely elevated because of the increase in preload.

Cardiothoracic surgery is not the treatment of choice as cardiopulmonary bypass is associated with a 50% risk of fetal mortality.

Rheumatic heart disease in pregnancy is common in developing countries and is increasing in the UK because of increased immigration.

30. A. Atrial fibrillation is uncommon in pregnancy. Management needs to focus on treating the arrhythmia and protection from thromboembolic events. Pregnancy is a hypercoagulable state, so full anticoagulation with low molecular weight heparin is recommended until 4 weeks after the restoration of sinus rhythm. If the patient is in AF for a short time this is not required, as with non-pregnant patients.

DC cardioversion is safe, but is not recommended unless the patient is compromised. The fetus should be monitored with CTG if this is required.

Many antiarrhthymics are relatively safe in pregnancy. Flecainide is FDA Category C (it is effective in medically cardioverting patients in AF and is often used to treat fetal arrhythmias). Beta-blockers can also be used (see Question 5). Digoxin is also Category C and is sometimes used for fetal treatment. The dose may need to be increased in pregnancy because of the increased glomerular filtration rate. Levels need to be checked in case of toxicity, which is dangerous for the fetus. Amiodarone is not safe in pregnancy (Category D). It causes fetal thyroid problems and intra-uterine growth retardation, and is teratogenic.

1. **A 40-year-old man is referred to the cardiology outpatient clinic from the ED where he had presented with a cough. A CXR had been performed and had demonstrated a widened mediastinum. A CT thorax was requested which demonstrated a 6.1 cm aneurysm in the ascending aorta. Therefore he was referred to you for further follow-up.**

   Which one of the following is true regarding the pathophysiology of aortic aneurysms?

   A. The presence of a bicuspid aortic valve doubles the risk of dissection
   B. Bicuspid aortic valves account for 2% of all dissections
   C. Dissection in patients with bicuspid aortic valves is due to post-stenotic dilatation of the ascending aorta
   D. Previous surgery accounts for 2–4% of aortic aneurysms
   E. Kawasaki syndrome tends to affect the coronary arteries of adults

2. **What is the likelihood that the man in Question 1, who does not have a known predisposition to dissection, will die within a year as a result of this aneurysm?**

   A. 4.1%
   B. 2%
   C. 10.8%
   D. 19.5%
   E. 6.6%

3. **With regard to the pathogenesis of aortic aneurysm, which one of the following is the most important factor?**

   A. Smoking
   B. Hypertension
   C. Cystic medial necrosis
   D. Type 2 diabetes mellitus
   E. Presence of FBN 1 gene

4. **In which one of the following conditions does cystic medial necrosis occur?**

    A. Marfan syndrome
    B. Ehlers–Danlos syndrome
    C. Bicuspid aortic valve
    D. Familial aortic dissection
    E. All of the above

5. **Which one of the following is true about the genetics of aortopathies?**

    A. Marfan syndrome is an X-linked recessive disorder
    B. Turner's syndrome is associated with congenital heart disease in 25% of cases
    C. All forms of Ehlers–Danlos syndrome have a risk of aortic aneurysm formation
    D. Two spot mutations in the fibrillin gene are known about
    E. The MMP-9 gene has been reported as being associated with thoraco-aortic aneurysms

6. **According to Laplace's law, a doubling of the radius results in:**

    A. Four times the circumferential wall stress
    B. Eight times the circumferential wall stress
    C. Twice the circumferential wall stress
    D. Half the circumferential wall stress
    E. Makes no difference to the circumferential wall stress as long as the pressure reduces by 20 mmHg

7. **A 33-year-old man is seen in the cardiology outpatient clinic. He is being followed up for aortic regurgitation. Which one of the following is true?**

    A. If he has Marfan syndrome and his aortic root measures 46 mm, he should be referred for aortic valve and root replacement
    B. If he has a bicuspid aortic valve and his aortic root measures 51 mm, he should be referred for aortic valve and root replacement
    C. If he has neither Marfan syndrome nor a bicuspid valve but his aortic root measures 57 mm, he should be referred for aortic valve and root replacement
    D. If he has neither Marfan syndrome nor a bicuspid aortic valve but his aortic root measures 47 mm and he has moderate AR with an end-diastolic dimension of 64 mm, he should be referred for an aortic valve and root replacement
    E. Answers A, B, and C correct

8. **You see a 60-year-old musician in the outpatient clinic who discharged himself 2 weeks previously following admission with a confirmed type B dissection of the aorta. He tells you that he doesn't want to take any medication as he prefers natural healing methods. His blood pressure is 180/90 mmHg. He asks you what the future holds for him off medication.**

    What can you tell him that the data suggest if he has no treatment?

    A. Approximately 1/6 (16%) are dead within a year and 1/5 (20%) die within 5 years
    B. Approximately 1/20 (5%) are dead within a year and 1/10 (10%) die within 5 years
    C. Approximately a third (33%) are dead within a year and half (50%) die within 5 years
    D. The type of tear in his aorta is not as serious as other types of tear and the herbal remedy *Echinacea* has been used successfully for this condition for hundreds of years in the Amazon delta
    E. None of the above are true

9. **Which one of the following statements regarding the choice of imaging in a patient with suspected acute type A aortic dissection is true?**

    A. A transthoracic echocardiogram is the first investigation of choice because of its availability and accuracy/ease of use/ability to assess the aorta and left ventricular function
    B. A plain chest radiograph with non-mediastinal widening is a typical finding in 50% of patients with aortic dissection
    C. A disadvantage of TOE is that part of the ascending aorta is obscured by the trachea
    D. Absence of ECG gating prevents accurate diagnosis of type A dissection in 35% of patients
    E. The presence of a Medtronic Surescan DDDR device is a good reason not to opt for MRI of the aorta

10. **Which one of the following is true regarding CT of the aorta?**

    A. Helical CT scanners of four detector rows currently offer the optimal possible data acquisition for state of the art reconstruction of the aorta
    B. ECG gating reduces motion artefact which is particularly useful when imaging the descending aorta
    C. If appropriately acquired, a CT of the aorta and a CT coronary angiogram can be performed in a single acquisition
    D. New-generation multidetector helical CT scanners show sensitivities up to 95% and specificities of 94%
    E. In aortic dissection the scan should continue to the coeliac axis

11. **You are called by the acute medicine registrar who wants advice on what to do with a normally fit and well patient admitted with aortic pain which appeared to be characteristic—sudden-onset sharp right paravertebral pain. The ECG demonstrated sinus rhythm with voltage criteria for LVH. The CXR was normal. A CT of the aorta was carried out and did not show an intimal tear or evidence of dissection. There was a comment about intramural haematoma proximal to the right subclavian artery.**

    What advice should you give him?

    A. It is analogous to haematoma that is laid down in areas of low flow in a large aneurysm and tends not to predict future events

    B. As long as the ascending aorta measures less than 6.0 cm discharge is safe pending follow-up in the outpatient clinic

    C. The presence of a penetrating ulcer measuring 1.1 × 1.1cm in the descending aorta would be a more concerning sign

    D. This should be treated as sign of impending rupture and the case should be discussed with the local cardiothoracic unit

    E. An MRI of the aorta is likely to improve the diagnostic yield and should be organized immediately

12. **Which one of the following is true regarding magnetic resonance imaging (MRI) of the aorta?**

    A. MR examinations last approximately 10 times longer than CT examinations

    B. A basic MR examination may include the following: black blood imaging; basic spin-echo sequences; non-contrast white blood imaging; contrast-enhanced MR angiography using gadolinium and phase-contrast imaging

    C. Black blood imaging is rarely used to evaluate aortic morphology

    D. Phase contrast imaging is performed to evaluate gradients across an area of stenosis

    E. Breath-holding is superior to ECG gating in preventing motion artefact

13. **A 35-year-old woman is referred to the outpatient clinic for assessment. She has a confirmed diagnosis of Marfan syndrome from childhood but failed to attend follow-up clinics when she was a teenager. She takes no regular medication. Her blood pressure is 134/76 mmHg. The ascending aorta measures 43 mm on CT. She wants to start a family.**

    What would you advise?

    A. Start a beta-blocker and screen regularly throughout pregnancy

    B. Withhold beta-blockade until she is pregnant; then start and monitor aortic root with transthoracic echocardiography at 12, 24, and 36 weeks

    C. Refer to a gynaecologist with an interest in fertility

    D. She has a 10% risk of dissection if she becomes pregnant and therefore aortic root replacement ± AVR should be considered; she should avoid becoming pregnant and contraception should be discussed

    E. Avoid beta-blockade as it has been shown to be deleterious in pregnancy; monitor carefully during pregnancy and have a low threshold for initiating antihypertensive treatment; recommend a vaginal delivery with a short second stage

14. **A 63-year-old male is admitted to the ED of a district general hospital with a short history of sudden-onset sharp back pain and collapse. On examination he appears unwell, flushed, and diaphoretic. His blood pressure is 85/68 mmHg, his heart rate is 126 bpm, and his JVP is elevated. The emergency doctors suspect an acute dissection of the thoracic aorta which is duly confirmed on CT and extends from the sinuses of Valsalva to the aortic arch. A moderate pericardial effusion is noted and you are called to 'drain this as the patient has cardiac tamponade'.**

    What should you do?

    A. Drain the effusion under direct ultrasound guidance and then refer the patient to the cardiothoracic unit for emergency surgery

    B. Transfer the patient urgently to the nearest cardiothoracic unit for emergency surgery

    C. Fluid resuscitate the patient on the CCU and re-echo him to assess for echocardiographic signs of tamponade

    D. Perform urgent transoesophageal echocardiography to assess the location of the dissection flap and determine the location of the presumed fistula from the aorta to the pericardium

    E. Perform a CT coronary angiogram to assess the need for revascularization

15. **How should an individual with blood pressure recordings of 161/97 mmHg be classified?**

    A. High normal

    B. Grade 1 hypertension

    C. Grade 2 hypertension

    D. Grade 3 hypertension

    E. Isolated systolic hypertension

16. **You have been referred a 65-year-old man whom the GP has been struggling to manage. For the last year his clinic blood pressure recordings have been persistently around 150/90 mmHg, but he claims to suffer from the 'white coat' phenomenon, with home recordings of around 135/90 mmHg which you are satisfied have been undertaken appropriately. He is otherwise healthy, having implemented dietary changes and increased his exercise over the last year, but smokes and intends to continue.**

    What do you recommend?

    A. A clinic recording, which if normal suggests no need for medical management and if >140/90 mmHg requires treatment

    B. A 24-hour ambulatory blood pressure monitor (ABPM)

    C. Salt restriction, exercise, and continued home monitoring

    D. Commencement of pharmacological treatment

    E. Home devices are not as reliable as a mercury sphygmomanometer; therefore the clinic measurements should be believed and treatment commenced

17. **A 55-year-old female inpatient has recently been diagnosed with a transient ischaemic attack (TIA), which was confirmed by cerebral MRI. Echocardiography and carotid ultrasound are essentially normal. Her blood pressure during admission is 130/80 mmHg.**

    What management do you suggest?

    A. Lifestyle changes
    B. Aspirin
    C. Aspirin and lifestyle changes
    D. Aspirin, lifestyle changes, and antihypertensive medication
    E. A bubble echocardiogram to look for a PFO

18. **You requested a 24-hour ambulatory blood pressure monitor to assess an individual's response to treatment. It has revealed an average daytime recording of 143/95 mmHg and a night-time average of 134/80 mmHg. He is aged 57, is non-diabetic, and has appropriately adjusted his lifestyle. Medication was commenced a year ago, and he has been on 5 mg of ramipril for 3 months with a recent tolerated mild cough, which may be unrelated.**

    What is the best treatment option?

    A. Review lifestyle modification, including weight loss
    B. Increase the ramipril to 7.5 mg
    C. Add an angiotensin receptor blocker
    D. Add a beta-blocker
    E. Add a calcium-channel antagonist

19. **According to the Joint British Society (JBS) Guidelines CVD risk model, every increase of 20/10 mmHg in blood pressure increases your 10-year CVD risk by a factor of:**

    A. 1.5
    B. 2
    C. 3
    D. 4
    E. 5

20. **Routine initial investigations in a 58-year-old patient with recently diagnosed Grade 3 hypertension should include all of the following, except:**

    A. Urinary albumin-to-creatinine ratio
    B. Serum creatinine and electrolytes
    C. Fasted blood glucose and lipids
    D. Fundoscopy
    E. Echocardiogram

21. **An overweight (BMI 35) 45-year old man has been referred for investigation of his high blood pressure (160/95 mmHg). He has no significant past medical or family history, but socially he consumes at least 15 pints of beer per week and smokes five cigarettes per day. A 24-hour urinary cortisol is raised and low-dose dexamethasone test is normal.**

    What is the appropriate management?

    A. Advise lifestyle changes including weight loss, exercise, and reduced alcohol intake
    B. A renal ultrasound
    C. A MIBI scan
    D. Refer to an endocrinologist
    E. Commence an ACE inhibitor

22. **A 16-year-old patient has been referred to you for investigation of a murmur. Auscultation reveals a mid-systolic murmur on the anterior chest. There does not appear to be a radiofemoral delay, but the recorded brachial blood pressure is 143/90 mmHg. There is a family history of premature stroke but no family history of kidney problems.**

    What would the best investigation be?

    A. Echocardiogram
    B. CT aorta
    C. Cardiac MRI
    D. Renal ultrasound
    E. Cerebral MRA

23. **A patient is followed up at a 6-week appointment following a primary percutaneous intervention for an anterior STEMI. An echocardiogram pre-discharge estimated overall LVEF as 40%. He is asymptomatic, compliant with all medications, and has no problems from side effects. His blood pressure is 95/70 mmHg, with no evidence of a postural drop, and his heart rate is 55 bpm. His GP has recently increased his medication to 5 mg bisoprolol and 7.5 mg ramipril.**

    What are your recommendations?

    A. Continue on the current regime
    B. Reduce ramipril to 5 mg
    C. Reduce bisoprolol to 2.5 mg
    D. Reduce both medications
    E. Repeat echocardiogram to assess the left ventricle and then decide the treatment regime

24. A 65-year-old hypertensive non-diabetic has an eGFR <40. Screening tests showed microalbuminuria and a normal renal ultrasound.

Which class of antihypertensive medication should you instigate?

A. ACE inhibitor

B. Beta-blocker

C. Calcium-channel blocker

D. Thiazide diuretic

E. Angiotensin receptor blocker

25. The side effects of the broad spectrum of calcium-channel blockers (CCBs) include the following, except:

A. Peripheral oedema

B. Gum hypertrophy

C. Dyslipidaemia

D. Negatively ionotropic

E. Negatively chronotropic

26. Which one of the following antihypertensive medications might you use to try and prevent new-onset atrial fibrillation?

A. Atenolol

B. Amlodopine

C. Bisoprolol

D. Digoxin

E. Losartan

27. The following is true of hypertension in the elderly, except:

A. There is an age-associated increase in systolic blood pressure (SBP)

B. There is decreased variability in blood pressure

C. Beta-blocker use should be limited to specific indications

D. There is good evidence for the treatment of hypertension in the very elderly (>80 years)

E. It is associated with vascular dementia and Alzheimer's disease

28. The following are risk factors for pre-eclampsia, except:

A. First pregnancy

B. Multiple pregnancies

C. Long-term partner

D. Pre-existing hypertension

E. Family history

29. Guidelines for the use of a statin in hypertension include the following, except:

A. Following a stroke

B. Type 2 diabetic diagnosed 11 years previously

C. Primary prevention with a CVD risk of 25%

D. Target levels of LDL <2 mmol/L and total cholesterol <4 mmol/L

E. Primary prevention in an 80-year-old

1. D. Bicuspid aortic valves have a 1% prevalence and are seen in 6–10% of all dissections. They have a ninefold higher risk of dissection. This is due to cystic medial degeneration, impaired fibrillin-1, and lymphocytic infiltration in the aortic wall, and not to post-stenotic dilatation of the ascending aorta as had initially been thought. Kawasaki syndrome causes circumscript aneurysm formation, classically in coronary arteries, and typically occurs in children.

2. C. The annual risk of complications of aortic aneurysms is related to aortic size. The risk of rupture and death increase significantly once aortic size increases above 6 cm (see Table 6.1).

The rate of thoracic aorta growth is 0.1 cm/year which is less than that of abdominal aortic aneurysms. The rate of growth is affected by aortic size and genetic disposition (e.g. Marfan syndrome). The 1-, 3-, and 5-year survivals for ascending thoracic aortic aneurysm are 65%, 36%, and 20%, respectively. Therefore surgical repair of ascending aortas is recommended when aortic size reaches 5.5 cm, or 4.5 cm if the patient has Marfan syndrome.

Table 6.1 Risk of rupture and death

Aortic size	Annual risk of rupture	Annual risk of death
>4cm	0.3%	4.6%
>5cm	1.7%	4.8%
>6cm	3.6%	10.8%

Adapted from Ellis PR, Cooley DA, Bakey ME, 'Clinical consideration and surgical treatment of annuloaortic ectasia', *J Thorac Cardiovasc Surg* 1961; **42**: 363–70, with kind permission of Elsevier.

3. B. The most common cause of aneurysm formation is atherosclerosis, primarily related to hypertension. Marfan syndrome is a significant risk factor for aneurysm formation and dissection, and therefore the threshold for treating these aneurysms is lower than in the non-Marfan population.

4. E. The aortic wall is composed of three layers—the adventitia, the media, and the intima. Aortic dissection occurs when these layers are interrupted, and blood flows typically between the media and adventitia. The media layer is composed of smooth muscle, collagen, and elastin, and thus conditions that affect the strength of this layer will predispose to aneurysm formation and dissection. Cystic medial necrosis occurs in Marfan syndrome, but it is also known to occur in other fibrillinopathies and is said to confer a more aggressive disease course. It occurs in 75% of patients with bicuspid aortic valve undergoing aortic valve surgery. Atherosclerosis results in reduced flow in the vasa vasorum and contributes to a cystic medial necrosis/degeneration-like condition.

5. E. Marfan syndrome has dominant inheritance. Having a first-degree relative with the condition is a major criterion in the Ghent nosology for the diagnosis of the condition. Fifty per cent of patients with Turner's syndrome have congenital cardiovascular disease, including bicuspid aortic valves, coarctation, and dilated ascending thoracic aorta. Routine screening for these pathologies has been advised by the ACC/AHA. Assessing aortic dilatation in patients with Turner's syndrome is difficult owing to their small stature. However, if the definition of a dilated ascending aorta is taken as a ratio of ascending to descending aortic diameters of >1.5:1, then 33% of patients with Turner's syndrome have dilated ascending aortas.
Only the vascular form or Ehlers–Danlos type IV is associated with aortic aneurysm formation. The disease is caused by defects in the gene that encodes the synthesis of collagen III (COL3A1 gene). It is dominantly inherited, although it can present sporadically, and is characterized by joint hypermobility, lax skin, and tissue friability.

125 spot mutations for the fibrillin gene are known. Matrix metalloproteinase is important in extracellular metabolism and increased expression of the gene encoding this has been seen in patients with thoracic aortic disease.

6. C.

$$W = Pr/2h$$

where W is circumferential wall stress, P is pressure, r is radius, and h is wall thickness

Given this, hypertension, aortic enlargement, and wall thinning are important factors in determining wall stress and therefore progression of aneurysms.

7. E. The ESC valvular heart disease guidelines 2012 recommend the cut-offs shown in Table 6.2 for aortic root and aortic valve replacement for patients with any severity of aortic regurgitation (AR).

Table 6.2 ESC Guidelines 2012

Maximum aortic root diameter	Class recommendation
≥45 mm for patients with Marfan syndrome	IC
≥50 mm for patients with bicuspid aortic valves	IIaC
≥55 mm for other patients	IIaC

Reproduced from 'Guidelines on the management of valvular heart disease', *Eur Heart J*, 2012; **33**: 2451–96, with permission of Oxford University Press.

8. A. Whilst type B dissections are not as lethal as type A dissections, they are associated with significant mortality if not treated appropriately. Mortality with no treatment is 11% at 1 month, 16% at 1 year, and 20% at 5 years. Approximately a third of survivors of acute dissection experience further dissection or rupture or will require surgery for aneurysm within 5 years. High-risk groups include the elderly, those with poorly controlled hypertension, the presence of a false lumen, larger aortic size, and Marfan syndrome.

At presentation, aggressive control of blood pressure to a target of 110 mmHg with IV beta-blockers and sodium nitroprusside infusions is recommended initially, and combinations of beta-blockers, ACE inhibitors, and other antihypertensive medications as outpatients with a less aggressive target of 135/80 mmHg. Maintaining a heart rate of <60 bpm has been shown to be beneficial in preventing complications in type B dissection.

Follow-up imaging, usually with CT or MRI, is recommended at 1, 3, 6, 9, and 12 months.

9. C.   Distal segments of the ascending aorta may not be well seen with TOE as the trachea and left main bronchus pass between the oesophagus and the aorta. TTE has a role in the acute setting but the sensitivity and specificity for accurate diagnosis remain low.

Routine chest radiographs are abnormal in 56% of patients with suspected aortic dissection. The sensitivity and specificity of the accuracy of CXR in acute aortic syndromes are 64% and 86%, respectively. These fall when pathology is confined to the ascending aorta. However, a completely normal chest radiograph reduces the likelihood of aortic dissection. In patients with aortic aneurysms, distinguishing a tortuous aorta from an aneurysm is difficult.

CT of the aorta is rapidly becoming the investigation of choice for diagnosing acute aortic dissection because of its availability and ease of use. ECG gating can help eliminate false-positive results (e.g. where an intimal flap is mistaken for pulsation artefact). As technology improves, one may anticipate accurate assessment of coronary involvement. Assessment of the aorta with MRI tends to be reserved for follow-up studies because of the time taken for the study. The Surescan device is an MRI-safe pacemaker.

10. C.   Most centres have at least a 16-detector row of CT scanners. There are reports of excellent quality images of coronary arteries using prospective gating in 320-detector row CT. ECG gating helps reduce motion artefacts, particularly in the ascending aorta and for the coronary arteries. The sensitivities of the new generation of multidetector CT scanners are nearing 100% and specificity is 98–99%. It is recommended to scan from the thoracic inlet to the pelvis, including the femoral and iliac arteries (http://circ.ahajournals.org/content/121/13/e266.full.pdf).

11. D.   Intramural haematoma is a precursor of classic dissection and is due to ruptured vasa vasorum into the medial layers and communication with the lumen in response to aortic wall infarction. It progresses to aortic dissection in up to 47% of cases but can also resorb. It should be treated surgically if found in the ascending aorta as medical management is associated with a significantly worse outcome (55% versus 8%). If it involves the descending aorta, watchful waiting may be appropriate, although there is a trend towards endovascular repair.

Aortic ulceration is also a precursor of dissection. However, these ulcers tend to be found in the descending aorta and if they measure more than 2 × 1 cm they should be treated with either surgery or endovascular repair.

12. D.   An MR examination takes two to four times longer than a CT examination. A comprehensive examination may include black blood imaging, basic spin-echo sequences, non-contrast white blood imaging, and contrast-enhanced MR. Black blood imaging is used to evaluate aortic anatomy and morphology. Whilst ECG gating increases acquisition times, it produces motion-free images of the aortic root and ascending aorta.

13. D.   Marfan syndrome is associated with a significantly increased risk of aortic aneurysm and dissection, and the normal threshold for aortic root replacement is 45 mm. If the aortic annulus and valves are affected, the patient may require aortic valve replacement as part of this, but otherwise the aortic valve is preserved where possible especially in a young woman in order to avoid long-term anticoagulation.

Pregnancy is associated with significant changes in physiology with an increase in plasma volume and stroke volume. Hormonal changes result in subtle changes in the composition of the aortic wall. This makes pregnancy a high-risk situation for a woman with Marfan syndrome especially, but not exclusively, if the aortic root is already dilated. Dissection tends to occur in the last trimester or early in the post-natal period. Therefore it is recommended that the aortic root is replaced when the maximal diameter reaches 40 mm in this situation.

There is a 1% risk of dissection during pregnancy if the aorta measures <40 mm and a 10% risk of dissection if the aorta measures >40 mm.

If vaginal delivery is planned the second stage should be short, and a caesarean section is recommended if the aorta measures >45 mm.

Expert consensus document on management of cardiovascular disease during pregnancy. *Eur Heart J*, 2003; **24**: 761–81.

14. B.   The priority is to transfer the patient to a cardiothoracic centre for urgent surgery. Drainage of the pericardial effusion will delay transfer and can accelerate bleeding and death.

Patients with suspected aortic dissection with hypotension must be carefully evaluated before volume is replaced. Hypotension or shock may be due to haemopericardium/pericardial tamponade, mediastinal bleeding, acute aortic insufficiency due to dilatation of the aortic annulus, aortic rupture, lactic acidosis, or spinal shock.

The mortality is high even with surgical repair—in-hospital mortality rates of 10% at day 1, 12% at day 2, and 20% at 2 weeks. Without surgical repair mortality is nearly 24% at day 1, 29% at day 2, and 50% at 2 weeks.

15. C.   Grade 2 (moderate) hypertension. The European Society of Hypertension and the World Health Organization–International Society of Hypertension guidelines classify blood pressure on clinic recordings. It is based on either systolic blood pressure (SBP) or diastolic blood pressure (DBP), and it is easier to remember the grades as follows:

1.   120/80 mmHg
2.   140/90 mmHg
3.   160/100 mmHg
4.   180/110 mmHg

16. D.   A 65-year-old non-diabetic male smoker will have a 10-year CVD risk of >20%. Home recordings are usually accurate and lower (10/5 mmHg) than clinic measurements where the white coat phenomenon does not apply. Treatment should be commenced if repeated home (or ambulatory average) measurements are >135/85 mmHg (Stage 1 hypertension) and, as the patient has already been trying lifestyle measures for over 3 months, pharmacological treatment should be recommended.

17. D.   Cryptogenic strokes or TIAs are 40% of cerebrovascular events. Patients are treated as for any cerebrovascular event, with aspirin 300 mg once daily for 2 weeks and then 75 mg once daily, lifestyle changes, and antihypertensive medication. Antihypertensive medication is recommended for normotensive and hypertensive individuals who have suffered a cardiovascular or cerebrovascular event or have established renal disease. PFOs are present in 30% of normal individuals, so should only be considered if there are no other obvious risk factors for a cardiovascular event.

18. E.   Optimal treated BP is <140/85 mmHg. SBP and DBP are equally important but SBP is more difficult to reduce. Whilst reassessing lifestyle changes is appropriate, most individuals in studies did not attain their target BP and required dual medication for the most effective treatment. Given the possibility of a side effect, increasing the ACE inhibitor is inappropriate and continuing monitoring would seem sensible. In a non-diabetic over 55 the British Hypertension Society would recommend either a calcium-channel blocker or a thiazide-like diuretic.

19. B. Blood pressure is one of the most preventable risk factors for cardiovascular disease. It is estimated that an increase of 20/10 mmHg in blood pressure doubles your CVD risk. The JBS CVD chart estimates the likelihood of a CVD event within 10 years. It is based on the Framingham risk, but uses CVD rather than coronary heart disease (CHD) as an endpoint. Framingham risk is based on a northern European male population aged 40–59, and thus is not accurate for all individuals.

20. E. Urinary albumin-to-creatinine ratio is a routine investigation for protein and blood to assess for target organ damage (TOD). Serum creatinine and electrolytes may help identify TOD and a possible cause of secondary hypertension (renal disease or Conn's syndrome). Fasting glucose and lipids help to stratify risk and will influence treatment. Fundoscopy is a simple examination that provides evidence of end-organ damage and can identify malignant hypertension. Echocardiogram is a useful measure of TOD (left ventricular hypertrophy) but is not a necessary initial examination.

21. A. This man has pseudo-Cushing's syndrome; a raised level of cortisol that can be found in obesity and during depression. High cortisol is confirmed most accurately by a 24-hour urine collection. A low-dose dexamethasone suppression test is used to determine whether the hypercortisolaemia is endogenous. If it is positive, a high-dose test is required to determine whether the source is adrenal or pituitary. A normal low-dose test makes pseudo-Cushing's syndrome a likely diagnosis, and this requires lifestyle intervention in the first instance.

22. C. Whilst an echocardiogram is not unreasonable, the clinical suspicion of aortic coarctation requires additional aortic imaging as most coarctations are post-ductal and thus difficult to visualize on echocardiography. CT aortography provides excellent images of the aorta, but it involves radiation. In a young individual who is likely to require repeated scans at follow-up a cardiac MRI which includes aortic imaging provides excellent image quality and diagnostic yield, and does not involve ionizing radiation. A renal ultrasound and cerebral MRA are more appropriate for individuals with adult polycystic kidney disease, which is an autosomal dominant condition that can also present as hypertension in this age group.

23. A. There is no evidence of a J-shaped curve in the treatment of hypertension in individuals with established coronary artery disease. The up-titration of medication was desirable and should be maintained in the absence of side effects.

24. A. The control of blood pressure and blocking of the renin–angiotensin system are essential to preserve renal function. The African American Study of Kidney Disease (AASK) showed that ACE inhibitors were better at slowing eGFR decline than beta-blockers or calcium-channel blockers. This is true of diabetic and non-diabetic patients, especially if there is evidence of proteinuria. Optimal BP control is <130/80 mmHg or <125/75 mmHg in the instance of proteinuria. It is likely that the benefits of renin–angiotensin blockage are additional to the benefits derived from absolute blood pressure reduction.

25. C. Peripheral oedema is caused by pre-capillary dilatation and, as with gum hypertrophy, occurs mostly in dihydropyridines. CCBs are negatively ionotropic and should be avoided in left ventricular dysfunction. Beta blockers rather than CCBs cause dyslipidaemia, reducing HDL and increasing triglycerides.

26. E. The Losartan Intervention for End Point Reduction in Hypertension (LIFE) study demonstrated a relative risk reduction of 33% versus atenolol. The impact of new-onset diabetes mellitus on cardiac outcomes in the Valsartan Antihypertensive Long-Term Use Evaluation (VALUE) trial population, showed a relative risk reduction of 23% versus amlodopine.

27. B. SBP increases with age whereas DBP plateaus at about age 60 resulting in an increased pulse pressure. The elderly have increased variability in their BP, and so several measurements should be made before diagnosis. Beta-blockers should be used in specific circumstances, such as with associated heart failure or CHD, as thiazide diuretics and ACE inhibitors have been shown to be more effective. The Hypertension in the Very Elderly Trial (HYVET) compared indapamide and perindopril treatment versus placebo for patients over the age of 80 with a SBP >160 mmHg. The treatment group had a significant reduction in stroke, mortality (stroke, cardiovascular, and all-cause), and heart failure.

28. C. Pre-eclampsia is hypertension in pregnancy associated with proteinuria. The blood pressure after 20 weeks is >140/90 mmHg, or a 30/15 mmHg increase from baseline, with 300 mg proteinuria in 24 hours. A new partner is one risk factor for the development of pre-eclampsia, which is believed to be secondary to the immunological basis of the illness. Other risk factors include idiopathic hypertension, obesity, chronic renal disease, and diabetes.

29. E. Statins should be used in all cases of secondary prevention in patients with hypertension, with target levels of LDL <2 mmol/L and total cholesterol <4 mmol/L or a 30% reduction. The primary prevention benefit of statins has been shown in trials of hypertensive patients down to a CVD risk level of 6%. This is not financially feasible; therefore the recommendation is for statin use if the CVD risk is ≥20% or established type 2 diabetes for more than 10 years. There is little evidence for the treatment of patients over 80 years old with statins.

1. **In which one of the following is ECG-gated coronary CT angiography not indicated?**
   A. Exclusion of significant coronary artery disease in patients with a low to intermediate pre-test probability of disease
   B. Diagnosis and delineation of the course of anomalous coronary arteries
   C. Following a failed catheter intubation of a coronary artery
   D. Diagnosis of significant coronary artery disease in patients with a high pre-test probability of disease
   E. Coronary artery bypass graft assessment

2. **Which one of the following patient characteristics is ideal for performance of a good quality coronary CT angiogram?**
   A. Atrial fibrillation with a low ventricular response
   B. High body mass index
   C. Contraindication to oral or IV beta-blockade
   D. Ability to breath hold for 2 seconds to 3 seconds maximum
   E. Ability to hold arms straight above the head

3. **Concerning heart rate in cardiac CT, which of the following statements is false?**
   A. On-table intravenous metoprolol may be administered
   B. 50–100 mg of oral metoprolol 2 hours prior to the study is recommended
   C. On-table oral beta-blocker is not useful
   D. Heart rate of ≤65 bpm is ideal
   E. Non-ionic low-osmolar intravenous contrast has been reported to have an antiarrhythmic effect on administration

4. **Concerning ionizing radiation in cardiac CT, which one of the following statements is true?**
   A. Cardiac CT is always performed in >2 mSv
   B. A patient with a low BMI will have a higher radiation dose
   C. Reducing the kilovoltage will reduce the radiation dose
   D. Prospective ECG gating gives a higher dose to the patient than retrospective ECG gating
   E. Calcium scoring has a higher radiation dose than coronary CT angiography

5. **Concerning coronary artery calcification, which one of the following statements is false?**
    A. The coronary calcium score is a good independent predictor of future cardiac events
    B. A normal coronary calcium score excludes flow-limiting coronary disease
    C. A high coronary calcium score will decrease the negative predictive value of coronary CT angiography
    D. Coronary calcium results in partial volume artefact
    E. The coronary calcium score correlates with total plaque burden

6. **Review the MPR images of a coronary artery shown in Figure 7.1.**

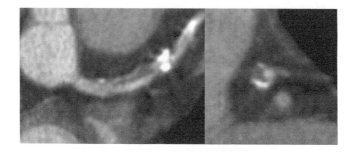

Figure 7.1

    Which one of the following do the images indicate?
    A. >50% stenosed mixed morphology plaque in the circumflex artery
    B. >50% stenosed mixed morphology plaque in the left anterior descending artery
    C. <50% stenosed mixed morphology plaque in the left anterior descending artery
    D. >50% stenosed non-calcified plaque in the first diagonal artery
    E. <50% stenosed mixed-morphology plaque in the first diagonal artery

7. **Concerning plaque characterization, which one of the following is false?**
    A. The Hounsfield attenuation value correlates closely with the characterization of predominantly fatty versus fibrous plaque
    B. The Hounsfield attenuation value correlates closely with the characterization of predominantly calcified versus non-calcified plaque
    C. CT plaque morphology has been closely correlated with intravascular ultrasound (IVUS)
    D. Vulnerable plaque cannot be identified using CT
    E. CT is the best non-invasive modality to diagnose preclinical coronary artery disease

8. **Concerning aortic valve disease, which one of the following statements is true?**

   A. The degree of aortic valve leaflet calcification, as quantified by CT, correlates closely with the severity of aortic stenosis
   B. Aortic valve planimetry measured using CT does not correlate well withTOE
   C. Severity of valve regurgitation can easily be assessed using cardiac CT
   D. Peri-prosthetic aortic valve replacement abscesses can be well delineated using CT
   E. Significant coronary artery disease cannot be reliably excluded prior to aortic valve replacement using CT

9. **A 55-year-old woman presents to the ED with recent-onset central chest pain presenting intermittently at rest, relieved by GTN, but not exacerbated by exertion. Her troponin I level and resting ECG are normal. She has no significant risk factors for coronary artery disease.**

   According to the NICE guidelines, what is the most appropriate subsequent management?

   A. Exercise treadmill test
   B. Stress perfusion imaging
   C. Catheter coronary angiography
   D. CT coronary angiography
   E. CT coronary calcium score

10. **A 78-year-old male ex-smoker was referred to the cardiology department with a history of COPD, dizziness, syncope, and exertional symptoms suggestive of angina. He had a suboptimal exercise tolerance test due to dyspnoea and could not tolerate dobutamine during stress echocardiography. He was referred for a cardiac CT.**

    A CT coronary calcium score was performed first and this is shown in Figure 7.2.

    According to NICE guidelines, what is the most appropriate next step in management?

    A. Proceed to CT coronary angiography
    B. Catheter coronary angiography
    C. Adenosine stress perfusion MRI
    D. Lung function tests
    E. Discharge with no further investigation

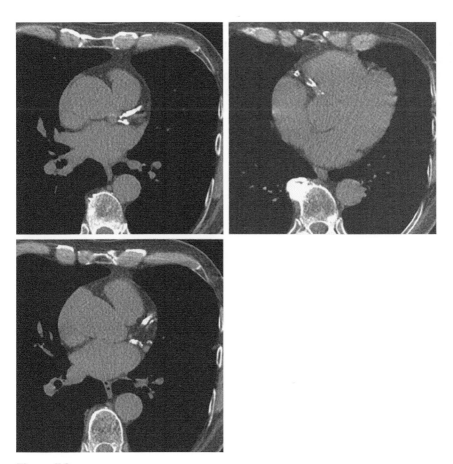

Figure 7.2

11. **A 45-year-old man presents with chest pain radiating to his left arm of duration 2 hours. There is no relevant past medical history. Troponin levels were measured at 1434 ng/L. The ECG is shown in Figure 7.3. 📹 Video 7.1 shows the CMR long-axis cine images and 📹 Video 7.2 shows the short-axis cine images. The late myocardial enhancement images are shown in Figure 7.4.**

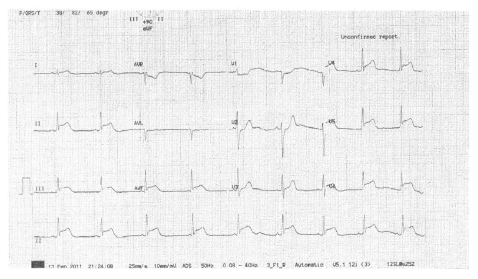

Figure 7.3

What is the diagnosis?

A. STEMI

B. Takotsubo

C. NSTEMI

D. Myocarditis

E. Hypertrophic cardiomyopathy

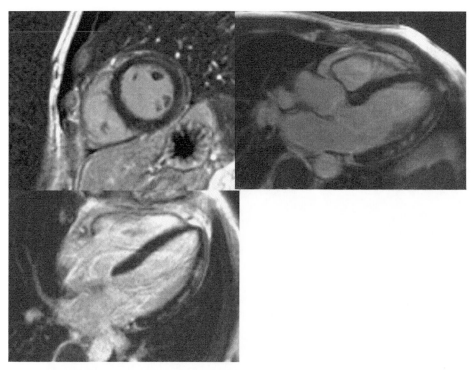

Figure 7.4

12. **A 65-year-old man presents with angina to the outpatient clinic. There is a past history of myocardial infarction 10 years earlier. You list him to have an angiogram. The angiogram demonstrates an occluded left anterior descending artery and a 90% stenosis of the right coronary artery. A CMR is requested to assess viability prior to any potential intervention. ▦ Video 7.3 shows the CMR long axis cines and ▦ Video 7.4 shows the short axis cines. The late myocardial enhancement is shown in Figure 7.5.**

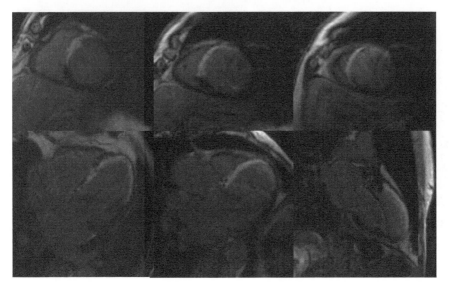

Figure 7.5

Which of the following statements is correct?

A. The LAD territory is non-viable

B. The entire lateral wall is infarcted

C. The RCA territory is non-viable

D. Both LAD and RCA territories show >50% wall-thickness infarction.

E. There is right ventricular infarction

13. **A 42-year-old man presents to the outpatient clinic with Canadian class 2 angina symptoms. His only risk factor is hypercholesterolaemia and he is on a statin. He is referred for an adenosine perfusion stress CMR to assess for inducible ischaemia. 📹 Video 7.5 shows the long-axis cines, 📹 Video 7.6 shows the short-axis cines, and 📹 Video 7.7 shows the perfusion images (stress, top row; rest, bottom row). The late myocardial enhancement is shown in Figure 7.6 in the four-chamber view (top left), three-chamber view (top right), and two-chamber view (bottom).**

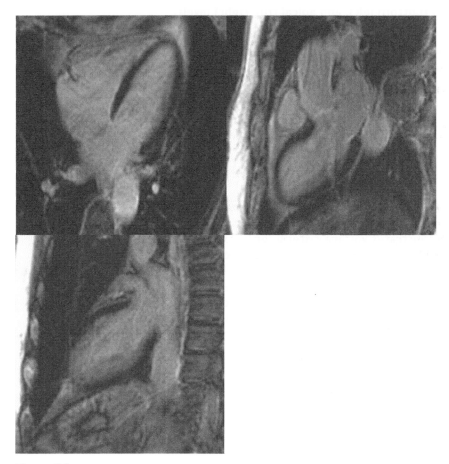

Figure 7.6

Which one of the following statements is correct?

A. There is myocardial infarction of the Cx territory

B. There is an inducible perfusion defect in the Cx territory

C. There is an inducible perfusion defect in the RCA territory

D. There is an inducible perfusion defect in the LAD and Cx territory

E. There is an inducible perfusion defect in the LAD territory

14. A 63-year-old man presents with a non ST-elevation acute coronary syndrome. His troponin is elevated at 650 ng/L. The ECG is unremarkable. He has a past medical history of familial hypercholesterolemia but is taking no medication. His cholesterol level is 11.3 mmol/L.

    He undergoes coronary angiography which reveals triple-vessel disease. A CMR is undertaken to assess myocardial viability. ⛑ Video 7.8 shows the long-axis cines, ⛑ Video 7.9 shows the short-axis cines, and ⛑ Video 7.10 shows the stress perfusion images at the basal (top left), mid (bottom left), and apical (top right) levels.

    The late myocardial enhancement images are shown in Figure 7.7 (top row, left to right: basal, mid, and apical short axis; bottom row, four-chamber view).

    Which of the following statements is correct?

    A. There is right ventricular infarction
    B. The Cx territory is viable
    C. The LAD territory is infarcted
    D. There is a significant pericardial effusion present
    E. The RCA territory is non-viable

15. A 73-year-old male presents with breathlessness on exertion. His current medication consists only of amlodipine 5 mg od. His ECG demonstrates voltage criteria for left ventricular hypertrophy. A TTE reveals LVH so he is referred for CMR. ⛑ Video 7.11 shows the long-axis cines and ⛑ Video 7.12 shows the short-axis cines. Figure 7.8 shows the late myocardial enhancement of the four-, three-, and two-chamber views (top row, left to right) and the short-axis views at the basal, mid, and apical levels (bottom row, left to right).

    What is the most likely diagnosis?

    A. hypertrophic cardiomyopathy
    B. amyloid
    C. hypertensive heart disease
    D. Fabry's disease
    E. None of the above

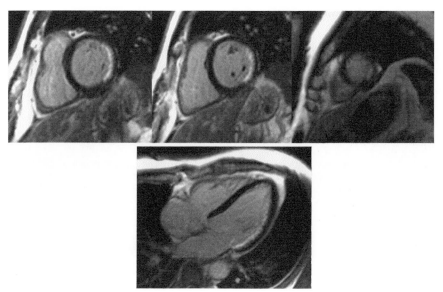

Figure 7.7

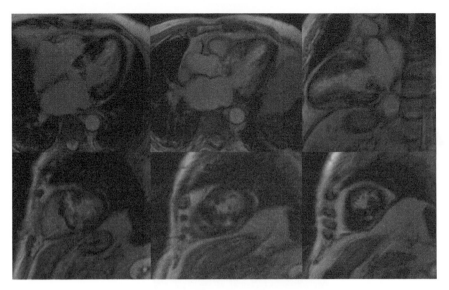

Figure 7.8

16. **A 66-year-old man presents to the outpatient clinic with breathlessness on exertion. He is a smoker with treated hypertension. A TTE reveals a dilated LV with overall moderate LV systolic dysfunction. He has a CMR to try to elucidate the cause of the LV systolic dysfunction. 📹 Video 7.13 shows the long-axis cines and 📹 Video 7.14 shows the short-axis cines. Figure 7.9 shows late myocardial enhancement following gadolinium in the four- and two-chamber views (top row) and at the basal, mid, and apical levels (bottom row, left to right).**

    What is the diagnosis?

    A. Dilated cardiomyopathy

    B. Anterior myocardial infarction

    C. Arrhythmogenic cardiomyopathy

    D. LV non-compaction

    E. Hypertrophic cardiomyopathy

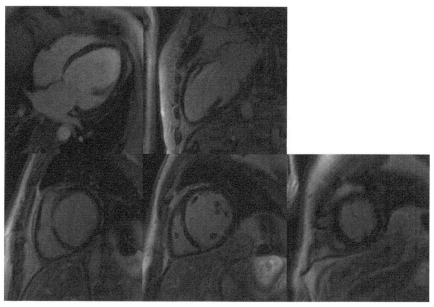

Figure 7.9

17. A 58-year-old man presents through the rapid access chest pain clinic with Canadian Class 3 angina. He is referred for adenosine stress perfusion CMR. 📹 **Video 7.15 shows the long-axis cines,** 📹 **Video 7.16 shows the short-axis cines, and** 📹 **Video 7.17 shows the perfusion images (stress, top row; rest, bottom row). Figure 7.10 shows the late myocardial enhancement.**

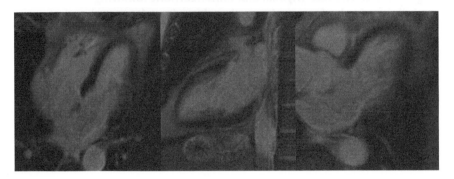

Figure 7.10

Which one of the following statements is correct?

A. There is no inducible perfusion defect

B. There is an inducible perfusion defect in the RCA territory

C. There is an inducible perfusion defect in the LCx territory

D. There is an inducible perfusion defect in the RCA and LCx territories

E. There is near full-thickness mid and apical inferior myocardial infarction

18. **You are asked to arrange a cardiac MRI to assess the left ventricular function of a patient following incomplete revascularization by percutaneous coronary intervention and stent implantation.**

    At what stage following the stent implantation is it safe to perform the scan?

    A. Immediately—there is no time limit
    B. Never—the static magnetic field will displace the bare metal stent
    C. Three months, to allow for endothelization of the stent struts
    D. After 4 weeks following cessation of clopidogrel
    E. None of the above

19. **Which one of the following is an absolute contraindication for an MRI scan?**

    A. An all-metal aortic valve replacement
    B. A St Jude mitral valve replacement
    C. A total hip replacement
    D. A bare metal stent in the LMS
    E. A cerebral aneurysm clip of unknown source

20. **A 60-year-old man presents with angina and heart failure. His estimated ejection fraction by echocardiography is 25%. An invasive coronary angiogram demonstrates widespread severe three-vessel coronary disease with good distal targets. A CMR study shows an ejection fraction of 22% and <25% myocardial wall thickness of hyper-enhancement in the mid and apical inferior segments.**

    Which one of the following statements is correct?

    A. The chance of functional recovery in the LAD territory is <20%
    B. The patient should not be offered revascularization because of the poor chance of functional and prognostic improvement
    C. The RCA territory has a >60% chance of functional recovery if revascularized
    D. He should be offered PCI to the RCA only
    E. His prognosis is better if he is treated medically than if he is completely revascularized

21. **A 55-year-old man presents with a 2-week history of dyspnoea following an episode of severe chest pain. An invasive coronary angiogram shows a 95% stenosis in the proximal LAD and an akinetic anterior wall. He is referred for a cardiac MRI viability study prior to percutaneous revascularization.**

    Which one of the following statements is correct?

    A. He should have a stent implanted anyway without the MRI
    B. 100% hyper-enhancement suggests that he should go forward for PCI to the LAD
    C. The scan should be done following the PCI
    D. Severe hypokinesis of the anterior wall suggest that the LAD territory is non-viable
    E. If a transmural infarct (100% enhancement) is present he should not have a PCI but should have medical therapy

22. **With regard to equilibrium radionuclide ventriculography (RNV), which one of the following is true?**
    A. Although RNV provides an accurate estimate of the LVEF it is poorly reproducible
    B. Only LVEF can be measured using RNV as the RV is too posterior and crescentic in shape to be imaged accurately
    C. RNV relies on the clear definition of the endocardial border and this is its main limitation in clinical practice
    D. Unlike myocardial perfusion scintigraphy (MPS), no radiation is used in RNV studies
    E. Poorly controlled atrial fibrillation limits the accuracy of an RNV study

23. **With regard to positron emission tomography (PET), which one of the following is true?**
    A. PET scanning is a cheap and widely available investigation
    B. PET compares poorly with CMR imaging when used to determine myocardial viability
    C. PET scanning uses thallium as the isotope of choice
    D. One of the major limitations of PET for cardiac perfusion has been that, until recently, the isotope needed to be produced on site in a cyclotron
    E. PET scanning utilizes changes in the metabolism of carbon to detect abnormalities of cardiac perfusion

24. **The following patients have sound evidence-based reasons to undergo an MPS study, based on the NICE 2010 guidelines for the assessment of chest pain.**

    Choose the single best answer.
    A. A woman age 60 years with an intermediate risk of cardiac pain
    B. A patient with chest pain and ST elevation on their ECG
    C. A bilateral amputee, with a recent MI and brittle asthma
    D. A patient with a massive pulmonary embolism in whom the RV strain is to be quantified
    E. A 62-year-old diabetic with unstable anginal symptoms

25. **A patient with severe LVSD and LBBB undergoes MPS. The following report is available to you in clinic. 'Adenosine stress (140 micrograms/kg/min) used over 6 minutes. 400 Mbq of ^{99m}Tc-sestamibi was injected after 4 minutes. Further dose of 800 MBq injected at rest. Line source attenuation corrected imaging also undertaken. Reduced septal counts noted on both studies. Probable anteroapical hypoperfusion noted on stress images. Normal counts elsewhere. Dilated LV cavity with global hypokinesia and LVEF 32%.'**

    Which one of the following statements is correct?
    A. This patient has undergone adequate stress
    B. This patient has a dilated cardiomyopathy
    C. Coronary angiography is not required
    D. There is evidence of a myocardial infarct
    E. Diaphragmatic attenuation accounts for some of the findings

26. **What would you do based on your interpretation of the MPS study shown in Figure 7.11?**

    A. Revascularization to LAD
    B. Revascularization to RCA
    C. DSE
    D. Medical therapy
    E. CTCA

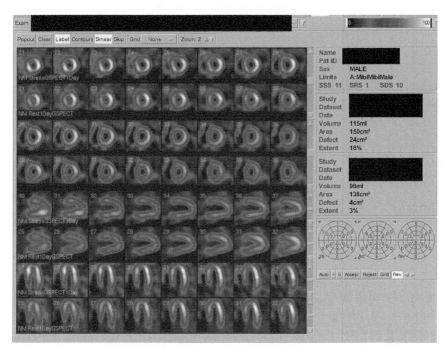

Figure 7.11 See also colour plate 1.

27. **This 45-year-old patient's coronary angiogram confirms a discrete mid-LMS lesion with a possible ostial RCA lesion following a recent admission with a minor troponin-positive episode of acute pulmonary oedema. Type 2 diabetes is the only risk factor. Echocardiography is difficult to assess because of obesity, but LV function is probably only mildy impaired.**

    How would you proceed based on the MPS shown in Figure 7.12?

    A. Optimize medical therapy
    B. Consider CABG
    C. Consider PCI LMS
    D. Refer for LVAD/transplant
    E. Refer for FFR or IVUS

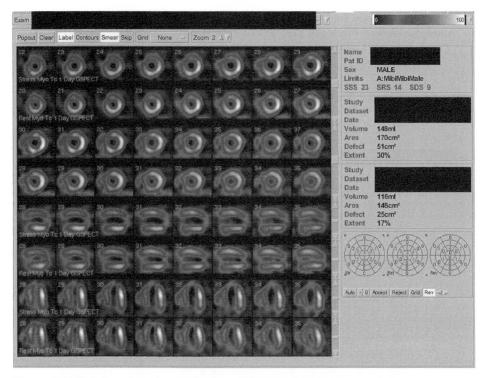

Figure 7.12 See also colour plate 2.

28. **This 75-year-old woman has undergone an MPS to risk stratify before a total hip replacement (Figure 7.13). Adenosine stress was performed without symptoms. Her past medical history includes hypertension, hypercholesterolaemia, and atrial fibrillation.**

   Which one of the following statements is true?

   A. The risk of future cardiac events is above normal (>1% p.a.)
   B. Repeat scanning is required in 2 years
   C. The patient is at low risk of a perioperative event
   D. Coronary angiography is required (invasive or CTCA)
   E. GI investigations are required

29. **Which one of the following statements about the study shown in Figure 7.14 is incorrect?**

   A. There is evidence of multi-vessel disease
   B. This is a prognostically high-risk scan
   C. There is inducible ischaemia in two territories
   D. Diaphragmatic attenuation is present
   E. Primary prevention ICD may be needed

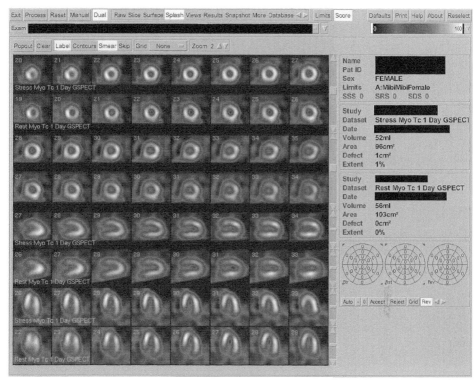

Figure 7.13 See also colour plate 3.

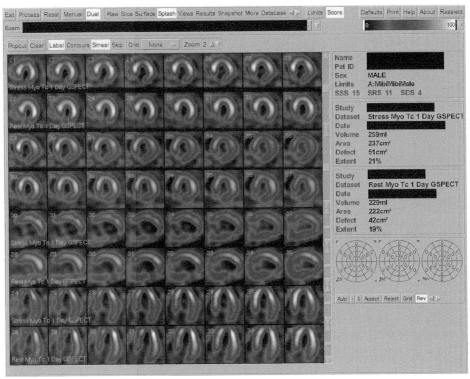

Figure 7.14 See also colour plate 4.

1. D. Coronary CT angiography has a very high (>99%) negative predictive value and therefore is an excellent tool for the exclusion of significant (>50% stenosis) coronary artery disease in patients with a low to intermediate risk of coronary artery disease.

Patients with a high pre-test probability of coronary artery disease often have a high coronary artery calcium burden which reduces the accuracy of CT angiography. This patient group is more likely to require coronary angiography.

Coronary CT angiography gives excellent anatomical delineation of the origins and course of the coronary arteries and therefore is extremely useful in the three-dimensional assessment of anomalous coronary arteries, including in the setting of failed intubation at catheter angiography.

Grafts may be occluded or difficult to intubate at catheter angiography, particularly when there is uncertainty over the details of the initial operation. Pre-procedural planning using CT may be considered. The accuracy of graft stenosis detection compared with catheter angiography is high.

Ollendorf D, Kuba M, Pearson S. The diagnostic Performance of Multi-slice Coronary Computed Tomographic Angiography: a Systematic Review. Journal of General Internal Medicine 2010; 1–10.

Stein P, Yaekoub A, Matta F, Sostman H. 64-Slice CT for Diagnosis of Coronary Artery Disease: A Systematic Review. The American Journal of Medicine 2008; 121: 715–25.

Abdulla J, Asferg C, Kofoed KF. Prognostic value of absence or presence of coronary artery disease determined by 64-slice computed tomography coronary angiography. A systematic review and meta-analysis. International Journal of Cardiovascular Imaging 2010; 1–8.

2. E. Many patient characteristics have an effect on the quality of a CT coronary angiogram. A slow (<65 bpm) regular heart rate is optimal for cardiac CT as a slow rate increases the length of diastole and thus increases the time when the heart is relatively still in which image acquisition can be performed. A regular heart rate with low respiratory variation is also important to minimize reconstruction or 'step' artefacts caused by ectopic or irregular beats. Thus, even with a slow ventricular rate, atrial fibrillation may significantly degrade image quality.

In view of the need for a slow heart rate, a contraindication to beta-blockers is not ideal, as this is the main pharmacological technique employed in cardiac CT for heart rate control; calcium-channel antagonists with a negatively chronotropic effect may be used as an alternative. Recent work on the use of sinus node blockers is under investigation.

Depending on the exact specification of the CT scanner and the field of view of image acquisition, the breath-hold time is 5–10 seconds. Thus if a patient can only breath-hold for 2 seconds, there is likely to be motion (respiratory artefact) which will degrade the image quality.

A cardiac CT is performed with the patient's arms extended above the head to ensure that there is no 'beam-hardening' artefact from the arms which reduces image quality.

3. E.

A heart rate of ≤65 bpm is ideal for cardiac CT (see Answer 2).Beta-blockers are the main pharmacological agents used for heart rate control in the context of cardiac CT, and metoprolol is commonly used.

A well-recognized protocol involves 50–100 mg oral metoprolol 2 hours prior to the scan. If this is insufficient, further metoprolol can be given intravenously on the table immediately prior to the scan, given its short onset and duration of action. Typically, 5 mg IV is given slowly, with pulse and blood pressure monitoring. This can be repeated with careful titration to an optimal heart rate. Oral metoprolol on the table is not useful given its long onset of action. Therefore it is ideal if patients referred for cardiac CT are optimally prepared with cardiology advice.

Contrast-induced nephropathy is a major cause of hospital-acquired acute renal failure, and its risk is significantly increased in patients with diabetes mellitus. The standard non-ionic low-osmolar contrast agents used routinely in contrast-enhanced CT are much safer and have fewer side effects than ionic low-osmolar agents. In addition, it has been reported that newer non-ionic iso-osmolar agents have less tachycardic and arrhythmic effects.

4. C.   Historically, cardiac CT has been recognized as a high-radiation investigation and this has been cited as an adverse reason for considering its routine use. Whilst the dose can be high, careful optimization of scanning parameters with aggressive ECG-gated dose-modulation techniques can result in cardiac CT being performed with a dose of <1 mSv.

Calcium scoring is a relatively low-dose study (currently <0.5 mSv) and is lower than a CT coronary angiogram.

Techniques to limit the radiation dose include reducing the kilovoltage (dose is proportional to kV^2) and limiting the scanned field of view. Prospective gating, in which the scan is limited to a fixed segment of the cardiac cycle (usually mid to late diastole), will also reduce the radiation dose compared with retrospective scanning, which acquires data (and therefore administers radiation) throughout the cardiac cycle. If a retrospective method of scanning is used, the dose can be minimized by using of ECG-gated dose modulation, with only a fraction of the maximal tube current (e.g. 4% or 20%) administered outside the useful diastolic reconstruction window.

The dose administered will increase with increasing BMI, as a higher kilovoltage (kV) and tube current (mA s) are required to penetrate an increased depth of tissue and maintain an adequate signal-to-noise ratio (good image quality).

5. B.   Coronary artery calcium scoring (CACS) was initially investigated using electron beam CT. Several scoring systems were devised, the most widely used being the Agatston score. This combines assessment of the volume and the density or mass of coronary calcium. Studies have shown that total coronary calcium is a good independent predictor of future cardiac events. The presence of coronary calcium confirms the presence of atheroma and correlates with the total plaque burden but does not always correlate with the location of a stenosis.

A coronary calcium score of zero is associated with a <1% risk of future coronary events. However, flow-limiting non-calcified atheroma is clearly not excluded and therefore clinical correlation is necessary.

A high coronary calcium score will decrease the negative predictive value and overall accuracy of a coronary CT angiogram, as calcium results in partial volume or blooming artefact in which dense structures can appear larger than their true size. This impairs visualization of the adjacent coronary lumen and can lead to an over- or underestimation of coronary stenosis when compared with catheter angiography.

Therefore CACS can be used as an important adjunct to the Framingham risk assessment and thereby significantly increase or decrease this risk.

6. B. The images show mixed-morphology plaque within the LAD causing a significant stenosis.

The proximal plaque is of predominantly lower attenuation, with mild calcification and a further heavily calcified plaque just distal to a tight stenosis. A corresponding orthogonal plane through the stenosis is shown. Non-calcified plaque may represent fatty or fibrous plaque, or often a combination of the two.

7. A. CT can accurately differentiate between calcified and non-calcified plaque on the basis of the Hounsfield unit attenuation value.

Studies have demonstrated a close correlation between plaque morphology as assessed on CT compared with IVUS, but CT cannot reliably differentiate lipid-rich from fibrous plaque given the significant overlap in appearance and limited spatial resolution.

In addition, CT cannot yet identify vulnerable or inflammatory plaque, although some work has been done on carotid arteries using nuclear medicine techniques.

CT is the best non-invasive modality for the detection of preclinical coronary artery disease as it delineates eccentric or shallow atheroma which has yet to cause significant luminal narrowing. In these cases, functional imaging in the form of stress MRI, stress echo, or nuclear myocardial perfusion would be negative because of the lack of ischaemia. IVUS is the reference standard for plaque detection and characterization, but has the disadvantage of being invasive and expensive.

Conventional catheter angiography is essentially a two-dimensional 'lumenogram'; an artery that has positively remodelled will have an atheromatous burden in the wall and therefore may look entirely normal.

8. D. Whilst the assessment of valvular heart disease is traditionally the domain of echocardiography, CT can provide useful information regarding valve anatomy and to a degree function.

Aortic valve planimetry has been shown to correlate closely with that of TOE.

The degree of aortic valve calcification has been shown to correlate with the severity of aortic stenosis, but the relationship is not a simple linear one and as the extent of calcification increases, the correlation becomes less reliable.

CT cannot directly or quantifiably assess valvular regurgitation. However, a number of indirect signs can be seen on CT, including a coaptation defect in the valve leaflets in diastole and a differential density of contrast in the left ventricle and left atrium in the presence of aortic regurgitation.

CT can be useful in the setting of aortic valve disease as it can be used to exclude significant coronary artery disease prior to aortic valve surgery and could save up to 50% of patients from needing preoperative catheter angiography.

In the setting of aortic valve endocarditis, the presence of vegetations or an associated aortic root abscess may make invasive catheter angiography high risk and technically challenging. In the setting of valvular infection, CT can also delineate aortic root abscess cavities and pseudo-aneurysm formation, providing important anatomical data prior to surgery.

Figure 7.15 (upper panel) shows a normal aortic valve (left) and a heavily calcified, thickened, and stenotic trileaflet aortic valve (right). The images in the lower panel show indirect signs of aortic valvular regurgitation with a coaptation defect (left) and differential contrast density in the left ventricle and left atrium (right).

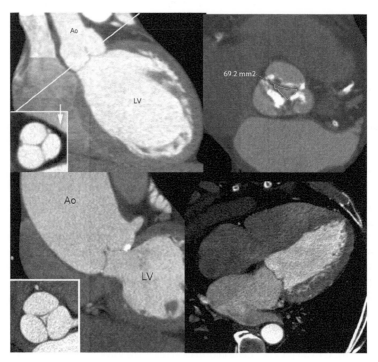

Figure 7.15

9. E. This patient has atypical angina. Given she has no risk factors for coronary artery disease, her pre-test probability of having coronary artery disease is 10%.

The NICE guidelines advise that the management of patients with a pre-test probability of coronary artery disease of 10–29% should have a CT calcium score as the first-line investigation.

NICE guidelines for chest pain of recent onset. Assessment and diagnosis of recent onset chest pain or discomfort of suspected cardiac origin, 2010. http://www.nice.org.uk/guidance/CG95.

10. B. The patient has a high pre-test probability of coronary artery disease and should ideally have gone directly to catheter coronary angiography. His calcium score was >3000.

NICE guidelines suggest that invasive catheter angiography should be offered to patients with a coronary calcium score of >400, if appropriate, and patients who are being considered for revascularization.

A heavy coronary calcium burden predicts significant coronary artery disease and reduces the accuracy of CT coronary angiography because of the partial volume ('blooming') artefact.

11. D. The ECG shows global ST elevation. The late gadolinium images show myocardial fibrosis in a non-ischaemic distribution (epicardial and mid-wall). Given the history, this would be consistent with acute myocarditis.

Ischaemic insults cause late myocardial enhancement to spread from the endocardium to the epicardium.

12. A. The septum and anterior wall is LAD territory. This is where there is late myocardial enhancement (white appearance of myocardium). The enhancement is >50% of the wall thickness; therefore the territory is classed as non-viable.

13. E. There is no late myocardial enhancement present on the late gadolinium images and therefore there is no myocardial infarction. There is an inducible perfusion defect in the anterior wall/septum (LAD territory).

14. B. There is late myocardial enhancement in the lateral wall which represents <50% wall thickness and therefore is viable. This distribution of late gadolinium enhancement is within the circumflex (Cx) territory.

15. A. There is asymmetrical LVH up to 20 mm with systolic anterior motion (SAM) at rest. There is replacement fibrosis of the regions of increased wall thickness. This is a case of hypertrophic cardiomyopathy.

16. A. Dilated cardiomyopathy (DCM). There are increased LV volumes with global, not regional, LV systolic dysfunction. There is a thin band on mid-wall myocardial late enhancement in the septum in keeping with DCM.

17. C. There is no late myocardial enhancement, and therefore no myocardial infarction. There is an inducible perfusion defect in the lateral wall which is LCx territory. The apical inferior wall can be supplied by a left dominant system.

18. A. The static magnetic field in an MRI scanner, although strong, would not create the shear forces necessary to displace a cardiac stent. There is no time limit for the examination, which can be performed safely during this hospital admission if necessary.

19. E. Most modern metallic valves are safe within the MRI enviroment but should be checked. It is generally recommended that the scan should be delayed following an orthopaedic procedure if possible, but if the clinical situation necessitates early scanning this has been reported as safe. Cerebral aneurysm clips are an absolute contraindication to MRI if there is no documentation of the type; this should be confirmed with the implanting centre and correspondence with the surgeon or radiologist involved.

Shellock FG, *Pocket guide to MRI procedures and metallic objects.* Philadelphia, PA: Lippincott–Williams & Wilkins, 2001.

20. C.   The patient has widespread coronary disease with good distal targets and viable myocardium; his prognosis would be improved with revascularization. There is no late gadolinium enhancement (LGE) in the LAD territory (meaning that there is >80% chance of functional recovery) and between zero and 25% LGE in the RCA territory (meaning that there is >60% chance of functional recovery).

21. E.   We do not know whether or not the anterior wall is viable from the information given; therefore the MRI scan is justified. A transmural infarct in the LAD territory with 100% hyper-enhancement suggests that this area is non-viable and would not improve with revascularization.

22. E.   RNV provides very reproducible data. New techniques allow the RVEF to be assessed. RNV is independent of endocardial border detection as it images radiolabelled red cell passage through the LV. It is a nuclear-based technique. AF will limit the accuracy, as gating will be less regular.

23. D.   This answer is correct, although rubidium-based isotopes may change this. PET remains a costly and specialist procedure. It uses glucose metabolism to detect abnormalities.

24. A.   Scenario B needs emergency angiography. Scenario C is unsuitable for current vasodilator stress agents; however, new selective A_{2A} agents which have much less bronchospasm (e.g. regadenoson) will soon be available. Scenario D should have echocardiography as the first line. Scenario E should be offered angiography in the first incidence.

25. A.   No information is given as to the size of the left ventricle. The report suggests ischaemia and therefore coronary angiography is required. The septal hypoperfusion is probably due to an LBBB artefact rather than a myocardial infarction. No inferior wall pathology is identified, which is sometimes masked by diaphragmatic attenuation.

26. A.   This is a high-risk study confirming significant anterior and anteroseptal ischaemia. There is a large ischaemic burden with LV cavity dilatation with stress. Revascularization to the LAD should be attempted.

27. C.   The LMS is flow limiting, as evidenced by the large area of anterior and septal ischaemia with stress-induced LV cavity dilatation. The apex is a small non-viable infarct. The RCA is not flow limiting and needs no further assessment.

28. B.   This is a normal low-risk scan. The 'warranty period' in a non-diabetic patient is approximately 7 years in the absence of new symptoms (less so in diabetics). Tracer activity is noted in the GI tract in the rest study. This is not a sign of GI pathology.

29. D.   The inferior wall demonstrates a predominantly non-viable infarct apart from the basal segment which is viable at rest and ischaemic with stress. The anterior and inferolateral walls demonstrate reversible ischaemia. The inferior septum is also infarcted (non-viable). This is a high-risk scan, and an ICD should be considered if LVEF is sufficiently impaired by the IHD.

1. **A 75-year-old man is referred for elective preoperative assessment. He is a smoker with a 40 pack-year history and diet-controlled diabetes. Baseline blood tests including renal function are normal.**

   Which one of the following factors would make you consider that further investigation was needed to assess his cardiac risk?

   A. His planned surgery was a total hip replacement
   B. His planned surgery was iliac aneurysm bypass surgery
   C. His age
   D. LVH on his resting ECG
   E. His history of diabetes

2. **You are asked to review a patient on a surgical ward who has been admitted for colonic surgery the next day to remove a tumour. You discover that she has a history of ischaemic heart disease and underwent elective PCI to the LAD 18 months previously. She is currently taking aspirin, ramipril, and simvastatin. She has a resting heart rate of 80 bpm in sinus rhythm. Her blood pressure is 105/80 mmHg. She is euvolaemic. The surgeon wishes to stop the aspirin prior to the surgery.**

   Which one of the following medication changes do you recommend?

   A. Stop aspirin, as the risks of postoperative bleeding outweigh the cardiac risks
   B. Start a beta-blocker in order to minimize her cardiac risks
   C. Stop the simvastatin, as statins are associated with an increased risk of cancer
   D. Continue aspirin despite the risks of bleeding
   E. Give a long-acting nitrate to help with perioperative ischaemia

3.   **You review a 45-year-old man in clinic. He is due to have surgery on his knee ligaments in 4 weeks' time. He is a smoker and has a strong family history of ischaemic heart disease. He is normotensive. He tells you that he is a keen swimmer and footballer, and injured his knee whilst training for a marathon recently. He currently finds it hard to walk unaided. Routine examination and resting ECG are normal.**

Which one of the following statements best describes your approach?

A. He needs no further assessment prior to surgery
B. He should have an exercise tolerance test
C. He should have a myocardial perfusion scan
D. He should have a stress echocardiogram
E. He should have a coronary angiogram

4.   **Which one of the following statements is not true regarding management of a pacemaker/implantable cardiac defibrillator during non-cardiac surgery?**

A. Avoid surgical diathermy/electrocautery where possible
B. If surgical diathermy/electrocautery is essential, monopolar surgical diathermy/ electrocautery is preferred
C. Programme an ICD prior to surgery to a 'monitor' only mode
D. Programme a pacemaker to avoid or minimize inappropriate inhibition, or high rate pacing through the 'tracking' of electrical interference
E. In emergency situations, consider positioning a clinical magnet over the ICD/pacemaker implant site to inhibit shock therapy (for ICDs) or cause asynchronous pacing (for pacemakers)

5.   **You are asked to review a 76-year-old man who has been admitted to a surgical ward with bowel obstruction. A CT scan suggests that a colonic malignancy is responsible. Urgent surgery is planned to relieve the obstruction. The anaesthetist has asked for your advice since the patient reports limiting angina and is not normally able to climb two flights of stairs without becoming breathless. He currently takes aspirin, ramipril, simvastatin, and bisoprolol.**

Your initial assessment concludes that he is currently free from angina and is euvolaemic with no signs of cardiac failure. His resting ECG demonstrates lateral T-wave inversion.

What would be your most likely response?

A. Surgery needs to be postponed until he has had an echocardiogram
B. Surgery needs to be postponed until he has had an exercise echocardiogram
C. Surgery needs to be postponed until he has a stress echocardiogram
D. Surgery should go ahead since his life would be at risk without it
E. His cardiac status is such that an operation is high risk and should never be considered

6. **You refer a patient for consideration of aortic valve replacement.**

   Which one of the following patients is least likely to need coronary angiography?
   A. A 38-year-old man who smokes 40 cigarettes a day
   B. A 42-year-old man with no cardiac risk factors
   C. A 48-year-old woman with diabetes
   D. A 48-year-old woman with no cardiac risk factors
   E. A 38-year-old man with diabetes

7. **A 75-year-old woman is admitted with an episode of unstable angina. She develops anterior T-wave inversion on her ECG and serum troponin is elevated. Initial treatment includes aspirin and clopidogrel. She undergoes coronary angiography which demonstrates a culprit lesion in the mid-course of the LAD. This is treated with a drug-eluting stent with good results. LV function is preserved.**

   Forty-eight hours post-procedure she has an episode of frank haematuria and then develops clot retention. The urology registrar reviews her and recommends stopping her antiplatelets.

   What is your response?
   A. Stop aspirin but continue clopidogrel—the benefits of aspirin are unproven
   B. Stop aspirin and clopidogrel—the risks from bleeding outweigh risks of a further coronary event
   C. Stop clopidogrel and continue aspirin—the half-life of clopidogrel is longer
   D. Stop neither—the risks of stent thrombosis outweigh the risks of bleeding
   E. Stop antiplatelets and replace with an IV heparin infusion since the effects are more predictable

8. **A 74-year-old woman undergoes emergency laparotomy after presenting with sepsis and peritonism. In the postoperative period you are asked to review her since she has developed atrial fibrillation and blood tests reveal a raised serum troponin.**

   Which one of the following is most likely to be the appropriate decision?
   A. The troponin elevation is of no significance in the postoperative period in someone who has been so unwell
   B. The troponin elevation is related to the atrial fibrillation but is not otherwise significant
   C. The troponin elevation indicates a myocardial infarction and she should undergo urgent angioplasty
   D. The troponin elevation indicates a worse perioperative prognosis but does not dictate the management
   E. The troponin elevation indicates myocardial ischaemia and she should be treated with dual-antiplatelet therapy

9. **A 54-year-old man is seen in the orthopaedic pre-assessment clinic. He has had stable angina and, in addition to medical therapy, has had disease in a dominant RCA treated with a zotarolimus-eluting stent 5 months previously. He is taking aspirin, clopidogrel, simvastatin, ramipril, and bisoprolol. He is free from angina, has a resting BP of 113/80 mmHg, and a heart rate of 48 bpm. His blood results are within normal limits, including a fasting total cholesterol of 3.2 mmol/L.**

    You are asked about changes to his medication.

    Which one of the following would you agree with?

    A. Stop aspirin and clopidogrel; the risks of bleeding outweigh the risks of stent thrombosis ase the angioplasty was >1 month ago

    B. Continue aspirin and clopidogrel; the risks of stent thrombosis outweigh the risks of bleeding even after >1 month

    C. Stop the beta-blocker because perioperative use is associated with increased stroke risk

    D. Stop the ramipril since he is hypotensive

    E. Stop the simvastatin since his lipid level is satisfactory

10. **You refer a patient for aortic valve replacement. Angiography demonstrates coronary disease.**

    In which one of the following situations would they also need CABG?

    A. An 80% lesion in the left anterior descending artery

    B. A 65% lesion in the circumflex artery

    C. A 55% lesion in the right coronary artery

    D. A 65% lesion on the left main stem

    E. A 45% lesion in the right coronary artery and a 55% lesion in the circumflex artery

11. **A 56-year-old woman is admitted for elective total knee replacement. She has severely limited mobility and surgery is expected to improve this dramatically.**

    She is known to have hypercholesterolaemia and hypertension. In addition to simvastatin and ramipril, she takes atenolol.

    In preparation for her surgery she is nil by mouth from midnight. She does not take any of her medications the following morning. Whilst waiting to transfer to surgery she develops chest pain, and an assessment by the ward doctor reveals that she has inferior ST depression on ECG. Subsequent serum troponin measurement is positive.

    Which one of the following therapies do you recommend?

    A. Restart her normal medication and proceed to surgery as planned

    B. Thrombolysis and heparin infusion

    C. Urgent angiography and balloon angioplasty

    D. Urgent angiography and bare metal stent angioplasty

    E. Urgent angiography and drug-eluting stent angioplasty

12. **A 67-year-old woman with rheumatic mitral valve disease has been under observation for many years. She is asymptomatic. Her most recent investigation reveals a normal-sized and well-functioning left ventricle. The mitral valve area is calculated as 1.3 cm^2. There is mild MR. The left atrium appears dilated. There is moderate TR with a calculated PA pressure of 45 mmHg.**

    She is due to undergo assessment for a total hip replacement. What recommendation can you give to the anaesthetist?

    A. No precautions are needed since the mitral stenosis is not severe
    B. She should not undergo non-cardiac surgery without mitral valve replacement
    C. The orthopaedic surgery can go ahead, but extra care should be taken with rhythm and rate control and with fluid balance
    D. She should not undergo non-cardiac surgery without mitral valvotomy
    E. Orthopaedic surgery can go ahead with antibiotic prophylaxis against endocarditis

13. **A 73-year-old man is referred for review in the cardiac outpatient clinic. He suffers from intermittent claudication and the vascular surgeon has recommended an aorto-bifemoral bypass graft. During the work-up it is discovered that he has an ejection systolic murmur and your opinion regarding operative fitness has been sought.**

    In your consultation you discover that he has no symptoms of chest pain or shortness of breath, and has never had a syncopal episode. Clinically, he has aortic stenosis. An echocardiogram is arranged and demonstrates a peak gradient of 85 mmHg.

    What is your recommendation regarding his fitness for the vascular surgery?

    A. He has moderate aortic stenosis, and the surgery can go ahead with no precautions
    B. He has severe aortic stenosis but no symptoms, and the surgery can go ahead with no precautions
    C. He has severe aortic stenosis and should be assessed for valve replacement before the vascular surgery can go ahead safely
    D. He has severe aortic stenosis and should have balloon valvuloplasty to enable safe vascular surgery
    E. He most likely has extensive arterial disease and, rather than surgery, should take aspirin and a statin

14. **You are asked to assess a patient prior to elective orthopaedic surgery. Which one of the following factors merits further risk assessment?**

    A Inability to climb two flights of stairs
    B Stable coronary disease
    C Tablet-controlled diabetes mellitus
    D Age >75 years
    E Atrial fibrillation

15. **Which one of the following sets of findings in patients undergoing non-cardiac surgery is associated with an increase in long-term mortality?**

    A. Pre-operative evidence of frequent ventricular premature beats or non-sustained VT
    B. Peri-operative small elevation in troponin level
    C. Post-operative temporary worsening of renal function
    D. B and C
    E. A, B, and C

16. **You are asked to see a 78-year-old man who is due to have elective abdominal aortic aneurysm repair surgery in 6 weeks. He reports exertional angina.**

    In addition to managing vascular risk factors, including continuing beta-blocker, ACE inhibitor, and statin, which one of the following is most appropriate?

    A. This is high-risk surgery; no further assessment will change management
    B. Recommend coronary angiography to establish intraoperative risk
    C. Recommend nuclear myocardial perfusion scan to establish intraoperative risk
    D. Recommend cardiac MRI to establish intraoperative risk
    E. Recommend coronary CT to establish intraoperative risk

17. **A 56-year-old woman is assessed for knee replacement surgery. She has a history of angina and had elective coronary angioplasty to a lesion in the right coronary artery 2 years previously. She is limited by arthritis but can climb two flights of stairs without difficulty. She reports no angina.**

    Which one of the following would you recommend to assess perioperative risk?

    A. She should have a stress echocardiogram
    B. She should have a bicycle stress test
    C. She does not need any cardiac testing
    D. She should have a nuclear perfusion scan
    E. She should have a cardiac MRI

18. **In which one of the following patients is carotid endarterectomy recommended?**
    A. A female with previous TIA and carotid stenosis 65%
    B. A female with no previous TIA/stroke and unilateral carotid stenosis 95%
    C. A male with no previous TIA/stroke and unilateral carotid stenosis 85%
    D. A male with recent TIA and 65% carotid stenosis
    E. A male with previous TIA and 75% carotid stenosis

19. **Which one of the following is used as a cardiac surgery risk score?**
    A. EuroSCORE
    B. TIMI score
    C. GRACE
    D. HASBLED
    E. Syntax

20. **Which one of the following factors does not add to the euroSCORE II risk?**
    A. Exertional angina
    B. Lung disease
    C. Myocardial infarction 61 days previously
    D. Insulin-controlled diabetes
    E. Pulmonary arterial systolic pressure of 45 mmHg

21. **EuroSCORE II can be used to predict operative risk for which one of the following procedures?**
    A. Three-vessel CABG plus surgical maze
    B. Isolated AVR
    C. VSD repair
    D. All of the above
    E. None of the above

22. **What does euroSCORE II estimate?**
    A. In-hospital mortality for patients undergoing CABG
    B. In-hospital mortality for patients undergoing valve surgery
    C. In-hospital mortality for patients undergoing cardiac surgery
    D. Mortality and morbidity for patients undergoing cardiac surgery
    E. Mortality and morbidity for patients undergoing valve surgery or transcatheter valve implantation

23. **The following conditions are considered to be clinical risk factors and independent clinical determinants of major peri-operative cardiac events, except:**

    A. History of ischaemic heart disease (angina or previous MI)
    B. History of cerebrovascular disease
    C. Heart failure
    D. Renal impairment (serum creatinine >170μmol/L or creatinine clearance <60mL/min)
    E. Type II diabetes

24. **A patient has been referred for CABG. He is concerned about complications and wants to know the risk of perioperative stroke.**

    What is the typical nationally reported risk?

    A. There is no risk since the aortic valve is not being replaced
    B. 1%
    C. 5%
    D. 10%
    E. If an off-pump procedure is performed, the risk can be as high as 7%

1. B. Vascular surgery, especially suprainguinal surgery, carries a perioperative risk of a cardiac event of >5%. High-risk surgery in the elective setting would mandate further assessment of risk, which may include non-invasive stress testing.

Orthopaedic surgery is considered intermediate risk surgery.

In the presence of the other individual factors, further investigation is not required since optimal medical therapy should be given. Additional risk assessment would not alter this management.

2. D. An antiplatelet agent should be continued, especially where coronary intervention has taken place. The risks of bleeding do not outweigh the risks of a coronary event in this circumstance.

Beta-blockers are helpful in reducing risk in the perioperative period but should be uptitrated slowly to avoid hypotension.

Statins are not proven to be associated with cancer. Abrupt withdrawal in the perioperative period might be harmful.

There is no evidence to support nitrates in this circumstance.

3. A. In low-risk surgery, regardless of the patient's risk factors, good functional status is an indicator of low cardiac risk. No specific investigation is needed but the opportunity should be taken to discuss future risk.

4. B. Bipolar surgical diathermy/electrocautery is preferred. The other statements are all recommended measures. The device should always be checked before and after surgery to ensure appropriate functioning.

5. D. Decisions regarding non-cardiac surgery should be made jointly by the surgeon, anaesthetist, and patient, with input from specialist teams. There is always a balance of benefits against risks. In this circumstance, surgery should not be postponed since the consequences of doing so might be life threatening. The results of further tests would not change this decision, but the patient should continue on his current medication.

6. D. Guidelines recommend angiography for everyone considered for valve surgery except men <40 years of age and premenopausal woman with no cardiac risk factors.

7. D. The risks of acute stent thrombosis are high unless full antiplatelet therapy is given. Neither agent alone is suitable. Heparin is not a substitute.

8. D. Troponins T or I are constituents of the myocontractile apparatus and act as sensitive biomarkers for cardiac ischaemia. Levels can be elevated in several clinical scenarios, and this should be seen as indicating a higher risk of morbidity and mortality rather than a diagnostic tool. In the perioperative patient there may be many cardiac and non-cardiac mechanisms for troponin release. Management should be based upon clinical assessment.

9. B. Drug-eluting stents carry a risk of stent thrombosis that continues out to 12 months, with reports of very late stent thrombosis beyond. Recommendations advise continuing dual-antiplatelet therapy for >12 months.

The POISE trial investigated the effect of a non-titrated dose of long-acting metoprolol in the perioperative period. Compared with placebo, there was a higher incidence of stroke in this group. However, several other trials suggest a protective benefit of beta-blockers, and the recommendation is to continue treatment.

NB: Currently emerging data suggest that everolimus and biolimus (with biodegradable polymers) eluting stents are safe with shorter durations of dual antiplatelets (3–6 months), but the question is based on current guidance.

10. A. Guidelines recommend combined surgery where there is a primary indication for valve surgery and a coronary stenosis ≥70%.

11. D. The risks of non-cardiac surgery within the next 6 weeks are significant and therefore, in the context of non-life-threatening orthopaedic symptoms, it should not proceed.

Thrombolysis is not a treatment for non-ST elevation MI. Angiography within 48 hours is indicated. Choice of stent use is a balance of many factors, but based on the information given in the question, a bare metal stent seems to be most appropriate since it will enable the discontinuation of dual-antiplatelet therapy after 1 month if necessary.

The safest option is not listed. That would be a full 12 months of dual-antiplatlet therapy following angioplasty with the most appropriate stent. However, it is clear that this patient has severely limiting symptoms which may need treatment within 12 months.

12. C. Non-cardiac surgery can be performed in asymptomatic patients with significant MS (<1.5 cm^2) and a systolic pulmonary arterial pressure <50mm Hg. Care needs to be taken to control heart rate and fluid balance. Development of atrial fibrillation can lead to serious deterioration. Open surgical repair or valvotomy is required for symptomatic patients or those with significant MS and elevated pulmonary artery pressures.

13. C. Aortic stenosis with a peak gradient of 85 mmHg is categorized as severe. Even without symptoms, valve replacement should be considered for high-risk non-cardiac surgery such as this vascular procedure. Balloon valvuloplasty may be an appropriate bridge to definitive treatment in the face of emergency non-cardiac surgery, but is not appropriate here.

This patient will most likely have extensive arterial disease, and needs aggressive secondary prevention, but an operation should not be denied on these grounds.

14. A. Inability to climb two flights of stairs represents a functional capacity <4 METs and requires further risk assessment. Although the other risk factors are relevant, they are each only minor predictors of perioperative risk. Optimal medical therapy would be recommended in any case.

15. D.   Peri-operative small elevations in troponin levels have been shown to be prognostically significant in high-risk and intermediate risk groups. Even in patients with end-stage renal disease, a minor troponin rise correlates with a worse prognosis compared to those with undetectable values.

Temporary worsening of renal function has also been shown to be associated with an increase in long-term mortality.

It is estimated that almost half of all high-risk patients undergoing non-cardiac surgery have frequent ventricular premature beats (VPBs) or non-sustained VT. There is no evidence that VPBs or non-sustained VTs alone are associated with a worse prognosis.

16. C.   Abdominal vascular surgery is high risk, but patient-related factors will adjust the risk further. Assessment is indicated if it will change management. Confirming the presence of coronary disease may result in preoperative revascularization, and will enable perioperative management to be tailored appropriately. The best evidence base in this circumstance is nuclear perfusion imaging. Although cardiac MRI may give complementary and even additional information, it is not currently supported by ESC guidelines. Coronary angiography should be recommended for the same indications as in a non-operative setting, but would not be the most appropriate answer here.

17. C.   Knee surgery is not high risk, but patient factors need to be considered. Although your patient has a history of IHD, her functional capacity is good (>4 METs indicated by ability to climb two flights of stairs) and she does not currently suffer from angina. Although there is good evidence that nuclear perfusion imaging can risk stratify preoperative patients, it is not necessary here. Other risk-stratification modalities may be useful, but are not recommended in ESC guidelines.

18. E.   The best evidence for revascularization is seen in patient E. A male with 50–69% stenosis and recent TIA might be recommended for revascularization. There is poor evidence to support revascularization in woman with previous TIA and <70% stenosis, or women with no previous TIA. Benefit is seen in men with no stroke/TIA where there is bilateral carotid stenosis >70%.

19. A.   The other risk scores are used in cardiology, but not specifically in cardiac surgery.

20. A.   Only CCS class 4 (rest) angina increases euroSCORE II risk. Presence of chronic lung disease (requiring long-term use of bronchodilators or steroids) and insulin-controlled diabetes contributes to risk. Myocardial infarction is considered recent and carries risk for up to 90 days. Even moderate pulmonary hypertension carries some risk.

21. D.   The updated euroSCORE II (2011) includes weighting for type of intervention, and can be used for isolated CABG, valve replacement, structural repair, maze, and tumour resection.

22. C. The updated euroSCORE II (2011) was derived from a large dataset where the primary outcome was mortality at the base hospital. It does not predict morbidity. EuroSCORE II provides weighting for the type of intervention, not just CABG.

23. E. Diabetes requiring insulin therapy is a risk factor/major determinant of peri-operative cardiac events.

The LEE index is considered to be one of the best currently available risk prediction indexes for non-cardiac surgery. The 5 independent clinical determinants of major peri-operative cardiac events are as listed in the question options. High risk type of surgery is the sixth factor that is included in the index. All factors contribute equally and the incidence of major cardiac complications is estimated at 0.4, 0.9, 7, and 11% in patients with an index of 0, 1, 2, and ≥3 points, respectively. The ESC guidelines recommend that the LEE index model applying these six different variables for perioperative cardiac risk be used.

The guidelines also use these 5 clinical risk factors to guide recommendations to initiate statin and beta-blocker therapy and to consider non-invasive testing.

24. B. Although the absolute risks will vary from unit to unit and from patient to patient, it is useful to know the typical risks of cardiac surgery. The Sixth National Adult Cardiac Surgical Database Report gives a typical risk of 1% for isolated CABG. An aortic valve replacement increases this risk to closer to 2%. Off-pump CABG avoids cardiopulmonary bypass and there is some evidence demonstrating a reduced risk of stroke, although since the patients selected for off-pump CABG differ in their risks, it is difficult to apply this to the whole population.

Poldermans et al. ESC guidelines for pre-operative cardiac risk assessment and perioperative cardiac management in non-cardiac surgery. EHJ 2009; 30: 2769–2812.

Boersma E, Kertai MD, Schouten O, et al. Perioperative cardiovascular mortality in noncardiac surgery: validation of the Lee cardiac risk index. Am J Med 2005; 118: 1134–41.

Biccard BM. Relationship between the inability to climb two flights of stairs and outcome after major non-cardiac surgery: implications for the pre-operative assessment of functional capacity. Anaesthesia 2005; 60: 588–93.

Lee TH, Marcantonio ER, Mangione CM, et al. Derivation and prospective validation of a simple index for prediction of cardiac risk of major noncardiac surgery. Circulation 1999; 100: 1043–9.

Vahanian et al. ESC guidelines for the management of valvular heart disease (version 2012). EHJ 2012; 33: 2451–96.

Fleisher LA, Beckman JA, Brown KA, et al. ACC/AHA 2007 Guidelines on Perioperative Cardiovascular Evaluation and Care for Noncardiac Surgery: Executive Summary: A Report of the American College of Cardiology/American Heart Association Task Force on Practice Guidelines (Writing Committee to Revise the 2002 Guidelines on Perioperative Cardiovascular Evaluation for Noncardiac Surgery): Developed in Collaboration With the American Society of Echocardiography, American Society of Nuclear Cardiology, Heart Rhythm Society, Society of Cardiovascular Anesthesiologists, Society for Cardiovascular Angiography and Interventions, Society for Vascular Medicine and Biology, and Society for Vascular Surgery. Circulation 2007; 116: 1971–96.

1. **A GP contacts you about a young woman in whom a formal diagnosis of pulmonary hypertension has been made. He has not yet received her discharge summary but tells you that she has had a 'range' of tests.**

   Which one of the following would have to have been true in order for the diagnosis to be made?

   A. An echocardiogram demonstrated a dilated right heart
   B. During an exercise echocardiogram, the estimated RV systolic pressure (derived from the jet of tricuspid regurgitation) was >30 mmHg at peak exercise
   C. A CT pulmonary angiogram demonstrated bilateral pulmonary emboli
   D. Mean pulmonary artery pressure at rest was ≥25 mmHg on a right heart catheterization
   E. During right heart catheterization, the pulmonary wedge pressure was normal

2. **You are asked by one of the echocardiography technicians to review an echocardiogram for an elderly patient who presents with breathlessness. Estimated RV systolic pressure, as judged by the velocity of the tricuspid regurgitant jet, is moderately elevated.**

   In terms of an aetiology of the pulmonary hypertension, which one of the following is true?

   A. The presence of normal atrial size in the setting of diabetes and hypertension, in particular, point to a left heart cause
   B. Lung disease is an uncommon cause
   C. Thrombus seen in the proximal pulmonary arteries means that chronic thromboembolic disease has to be the explanation for the pulmonary hypertension
   D. The fact that the referral has come from a rheumatologist helps shed light on the cause
   E. Echocardiographic evidence of an old myocardial infarction is unlikely to be related

3. **You admit a middle-aged woman on the acute take who has been investigated for breathlessness for several years. Pulmonary hypertension is suspected.**

   What should you do?

   A. Start sildenafil
   B. Give warfarin in patients with pulmonary hypertension but no thromboembolic disease
   C. Withhold diuretics in the setting of overt right heart failure
   D. Give an ACE inhibitor to benefit the right ventricle
   E. Give an angiotensin receptor blocker

4. **A 70-year-old woman with a history of proven recurrent pulmonary emboli but no other comorbidities presents with breathlessness over a number of months. She is in NYHA class III. Her INR has been within the therapeutic range. Serial echocardiograms demonstrate persistent features of pulmonary hypertension.**

   Which one of the following is the most important measure?

   A. Persist with warfarin; the clot will resolve eventually
   B. Immediately work up for advanced oral therapies
   C. Refer her for consideration of pulmonary end-arterectomy
   D. Change her anticoagulant
   E. Refer her for a balloon atrial septostomy

5. **You have been contacted by the infectious diseases team about a man with HIV who has become progressively more breathless over a series of months. He has had a CT pulmonary angiogram which has excluded clots. You discuss the scan with the radiologist.**

   What else would you like to know about the CT?

   A. The size of the right ventricle—if it is normal, this excludes pulmonary hypertension as a cause for his symptoms
   B. The position of the interventricular septum as this indicates the balance of pressures between right and left atrium
   C. Whether there is reflux of contrast into the superior vena cava since this suggests elevated right atrial pressures
   D. The size of the pulmonary arteries—if these are dilated, it suggests that pulmonary hypertension might be present
   E. A pericardial effusion is not in keeping with pulmonary hypertension and should trigger a search for malignancy

6. **You are managing a patient admitted with worsening heart failure symptoms. She has been diagnosed with idiopathic pulmonary arterial hypertension and receives continuous IV epoprostenol.**

   Which one of the following is true?

   A. An interruption to the infusion can be tolerated for hours

   B. Redness around the line infusion site is expected

   C. Treatment with this agent would have been started when the patient was in NYHA class III or IV

   D. This treatment will not be used in combination with other advanced therapies

   E. Ramipril should be considered if the patient is not already on it

7. **You are invited by your consultant to study data recorded from right heart catheterization.**

   Which one of the following is true?

   A. The transpulmonary gradient is the difference between mean pulmonary artery pressure (mPAP) and mean pulmonary wedge pressure (mPWP)

   B. The pulmonary vascular resistance is the transpulmonary gradient (TPG) multiplied by the cardiac output (CO)

   C. Left atrial hypertension is reflected by a pulmonary wedge pressure >20 mmHg

   D. A positive pulmonary vasodilator test is indicative of a patient who will always respond to calcium-channel blockade

   E. Adenosine is used to assess vasodilatation response

8. **Which one of the following factors would worry you about a patient with pulmonary arterial hypertension?**

   A. A six-minute walk distance >380 m

   B. Static symptoms

   C. $MV_{O_2} < 12$ mL/min/kg

   D. Normal BNP levels

   E. Right atrial pressure (RAP) <10 mmHg

9. **Concerning the treatment of pulmonary hypertension:**

   A. Pulmonary transplant is never considered

   B. Sildenafil is recommended as a treatment for patients with left heart failure

   C. A majority of patients are on calcium-channel blockade

   D. Sildenafil was originally tried as an anti-anginal

   E. Prostanoid preparations are only intravenous

10. **With respect to pulmonary hypertension patients with congenital heart disease:**

    A. Pregnancy is well tolerated, making counselling on the topic unnecessary

    B. Venesection is recommended to reduce hyperviscosity relating to high hematocrit

    C. Eisenmenger syndrome describes reversal of a right to left shunt due to the development of pulmonary hypertension

    D. Transthoracic echocardiography inadequately images the upper septum and so sinus venous defects may be missed

    E. The six-minute walk test is an infallible measure of disease severity

11. **You are reviewing a 42-year-old man in the outpatient clinic who is under follow-up for recurrent troublesome attacks of acute pericarditis. He has had 16 episodes of pericarditis which initially followed a viral illness. No underlying systemic cause has been found despite extensive investigations. The episodes are associated with small- to moderate-sized pericardial effusions. Initially, the episodes respond well to systemic steroids; however, he has troublesome steroid side effects. On weaning the steroids with appropriate colchicine cover, the episodes recur.**

What is the best option with regard to management?

A. Plan to continue steroids long term at a lower dose as dual therapy with colchicine; appropriate bone protection should be given

B. Leave him off treatment and advise him to return immediately to the ED for early pericardiocentesis with topical high-dose steroid administration if his symptoms recur

C. Liaise with the rheumatological team regarding administration of immunosuppressant therapy as the most likely underlying pathological process is one of autoimmunity

D. Refer to cardiothoracic surgeons for consideration of total pericardiectomy

E. Continue to manage episodes with steroids and colchicine and monitor with annual echocardiograms for development of constrictive pericarditis

1. D. Pulmonary hypertension (PH) is defined as mPAP ≥25 mmHg *at rest* using invasive measurements made during right heart catheterization. Values during exercise are currently excluded from this definition. In PH, a normal wedge pressure suggests that the cause is not left heart disease. A normal-sized right heart does not exclude PH. Conversely, the presence of pulmonary emboli does not mean that the pulmonary artery pressure will definitely be elevated.

2. D. The echocardiogram in PH can be instructive as to the underlying aetiology. Left heart disease and lung disease/hypoxia are common causes. Left atrial dilatation is a red flag for left heart disease. Be mindful of systemic disease processes such as connective tissue disease which can underlie pulmonary arterial hypertension. Proximal pulmonary artery thrombus can form *in situ* due to sluggish flow when the pulmonary arteries are dilated, especially in patients with Eisenmenger syndrome.

3. B. Routine therapies given for patients with PH include warfarin (even if the underlying aetiology is not chronic thromboembolic disease) to attenuate the risk of *in situ* thrombus formation. Diuretics are given in those with overt right heart failure. Involvement by a specialist centre is essential. Advanced drug therapies should not be started without specialist input as they can be harmful. ACE inhibitors are not indicated for right heart failure.

4. C. This description fits with a diagnosis of chronic thromboembolic PH (CTEPH). In those patients with CTEPH in whom anticoagulation at therapeutic levels has proved ineffective at bringing down pulmonary pressures, consideration should be given to surgery with pulmonary end-arterectomy. This procedure can be curative in carefully selected patients. Advanced therapies can be considered if the patient is felt to be inoperable. Balloon atrial septostomy, which permits the right heart to vent into the left atrium, is used infrequently in selected patients with refractory syncope and heart failure.

5. D. CT can provide important information in addition to the presence or absence of pulmonary emboli. An enlarged right ventricle (though it can be normally sized), right atrium, and pulmonary arteries are all features of PH. Contrast reflux into the inferior vena cava implies tricuspid regurgitation and increased right atrial pressure. The latter is also indicated when the right atrium is dilated. The position of the interventricular septum and the interatrial septum reflects the balance of pressures between the ventricles and atria, respectively.

6. C. IV epoprostenol addresses the altered prostacylin pathway in pulmonary arterial hypertension. It is the only therapy in which mortality benefit has been demonstrated using a randomized controlled trial. It is indicated when patients are in WHO-FC III and are deteriorating or are in WHO-FC IV, and is often used in combination with other therapies. Specialist nursing input is required. The infusion should never be interrupted and pain/redness around the line entry site suggests infection which requires immediate attention. Spironolactone is an important diuretic for those in overt right heart failure.

7. A. Transpulmonary gradient (TPG) is given by mPAP − mPWP and is normally <12 mmHg. Pulmonary vascular resistance is given by TPG divided by CO. A PWP >15 mmHg indicates left atrial hypertension.

A vasodilator challenge is performed with inhaled nitric oxide to identify the small subset of patients with pulmonary arterial hypertension who will benefit from long-term calcium-channel blockade. A portion of those with an initially positive response (↓mPAP ≥10 mmHg to ≤40 mmHg with ↓/normal CO) will become refractory to vasodilator provocation (and therefore calcium-channel blockade) in the future.

8. C. It is key to identify the sickest patients in order to prioritize treatments. The following are recommended features which can be used to prognosticate: clinical evidence of RV failure, rapidly progressive symptoms, six-minute walk distance <380 m, peak oxygen consumption <12 mL/min/kg, high/rising BNP levels, pericardial effusion or TAPSE <1.5 cm, RAP >10 mmHg, cardiac index <2.1 L/min/m^2.

9. D. Sildenafil, which was originally developed as an anti-anginal before being used for erectile dysfunction, can be harmful in patients with PH secondary to left heart disease. Prostanoids are available in subcutaneous and inhaled preparations. Since only a minority of patients with pulmonary arterial hypertension respond to a vasodilator challenge (not all of whom will maintain this response), relatively few are on calcium-channel blockade. Transplant is considered for eligible patients.

10. D. Pulmonary hypertension is an important complication in congenital heart disease. At the most extreme end of the spectrum is Eisenmenger syndrome, defined by reversal of a left to right shunt due to the development of pulmonary hypertension. Venesection for patients with Eisenmenger syndrome is now avoided. A sinus venosus defect (and aberrant pulmonary venous drainage) should be considered in patients with a dilated right heart and PH but no other explanation. A transoesophageal echocardiogram can visualize the upper inter-atrial septum well. The development of PAH can make pregnancy hazardous, and the oral contraceptive pill can interact with bosentan. Therefore family planning is vital. The six-minute walk test has recognized limitations. Therefore a number of factors are looked at when trying to prognosticate.

11. D. This is a case of idiopathic pericarditis with characteristic recurrences on steroid withdrawal. Surgical pericardiectomy has been shown to alleviate the disorder and should be considered in cases of troublesome recurrent disease. There is a risk of failure to resolve symptoms if there is residual pericardial tissue postoperatively. In addition, recurrent disease can occur in the visceral pericardium, which cannot be stripped surgically.

1. You are seeing a 24-year-old man (A) referred by his GP as he is concerned about his risk of Fabry disease which runs in his family, as shown in the pedigree in Figure 10.1.

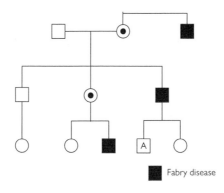

Fabry disease

Figure 10.1

What is his risk of having the condition?

A. 0
B. 1 in 8
C. 1 in 4
D. 1 in 2
E. 1

2. You are looking after a 38-year-old man on the ward who was admitted with a STEMI and treated with PCI. His total cholesterol has been found to be 11.8 mmol/L with LDL 7.3 mmol/L, and he has corneal arcus, tendon xanthomata, and a paternal family history of premature cardiovascular disease.

What is the most likely causative gene?

A. Proprotein convertase subtilisin-kexin type 9 (*PCSK9*)
B. Low-density lipoprotein receptor (*LDLR*)
C. Apolipoprotein B-100 (*APOB*)
D. Sterol 27-hydroxylase (*CYP27A1*)
E. Low-density lipoprotein receptor adaptor protein 1 (*FHCB2/ARH*)

3. **You are seeing a 28-year-old man in clinic. He has long QT sydrome due to a mutation in the *KCNH2* gene. He has two sons and a daughter. One son and his daughter have been tested and found to have the same mutation as him.**

   What is the chance that his younger son also has this mutation?

   A. 0
   B. 1/3
   C. 1/2
   D. 2/3
   E. 1

4. **You are referred a 28-year-old man following a private medical assessment which included echocardiography. This is reported as showing increased trabeculation.**

   Which one of the following would not be associated with this being a pathological finding?

   A. The trabeculations are predominantly in the right ventricle
   B. He has exertional dyspnoea
   C. The ratio of trabeculated to non-trabeculated myocardium is 2.8
   D. There is an ejection fraction of 38%
   E. His father died of a cerebrovascular accident

5. **You are reviewing a 17-year-old girl who has been transferred from the paediatric service. She had pulmonary stenosis treated in infancy. She has learning difficulties and facial dysmorphism.**

   Which one of the following is *not* in the differential diagnosis?

   A. Holt–Oram syndrome
   B. Noonan syndrome
   C. 22q11 microdeletion syndrome
   D. Loeys–Dietz syndrome
   E. Costello syndrome

6. **You see a 34-year-old man for his annual review for hypertrophic cardiomyopathy.**

   Which one of the following is *not* considered a risk factor for sudden death?

   A. Non-sustained VT (rate 200 bpm) on 48-hour Holter monitor
   B. Two syncopal episodes in childhood
   C. A history of sudden death in his paternal uncle at age 24 years
   D. Blood pressure drop of 40 mmHg on treadmill testing
   E. Asymmetrical septal hypertrophy up to 34 mm

7. You are looking after a 34-year-old man as an inpatient after admission with a type **A** thoracic aortic dissection.

    Which one of the following would make you think that Loeys–Dietz syndrome is a more likely cause than Marfan syndrome?

    A. Dural ectasia
    B. Ectopia lentis
    C. Myopia
    D. Widely spaced eyes
    E. Mitral valve prolapse

8. **Which one of the following genes is not associated with aortic disease?**

    A. Fibrillin
    B. *MYH11*
    C. *TGFBR1*
    D. Elastin
    E. *KCNH2*

9. **You see a family in clinic who have a dominantly inherited *SCN5A* (cardiac sodium channel) mutation. Which one of the following cardiac problems would you not expect to be due to this?**

    A. Brugada syndrome
    B. Long QT syndrome
    C. Atrial fibrillation
    D. Sick sinus syndrome
    E. Catecholaminergic paroxysmal ventricular tachycardia

10. You are seeing a 34-year-old man with left ventricular hypertrophy (LVH). He has a family history of LVH, as shown in the pedigree in Figure 10.2.

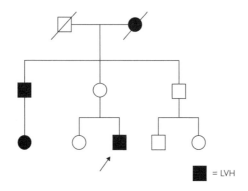

= LVH

Figure 10.2

Which one of the following is the most appropriate differential diagnosis of the cause?

A. Sarcomere gene mutation, mitochondrial DNA mutation, or Fabry disease

B. Sarcomere gene mutation or laminopathy

C. Sarcomere gene mutation or Fabry disease

D. Fabry disease

E. Sarcomere gene mutation

11. Which one of the following is not correct regarding the SCORE risk charts?

A. The UK is considered a low-risk population

B. Estimates the 10-year risk of a first fatal atherosclerotic event

C. Total CVD event risk can be estimated by multiplying by 3

D. Diabetes is part of the scoring system

E. >10% = very high risk, 5–10% = high risk, 1–5% = moderate risk, and <1% = low risk

12. A type 2 diabetic patient has proven microalbuminaemia. The fasting lipid profile is:

TC   4.0
LDL   1.9

What do you recommend regarding lipid control?

A. Continue current lifestyle regime

B. Escalation of lifestyle modification

C. If SCORE risk >10% start a statin—otherwise continue with lifestyle modification

D. Statin therapy

E. Increase oily fish consumption

13. **A patient who has recently had a myocardial infarction asks you about their target cholesterol.**

    What do you recommend?

    A. LDL-C <1.8
    B. LDL-C <2.5
    C. TC <5.0 (LDL-C <3.0)
    D. TC <4.0 (LDL-C <2.0)
    E. LDL-C <2.0, HDL-C >2.0

14. **A patient 12 months post myocardial infarction is complaining of muscle aches. The GP highlights that this may be due to simvastatin 80 mg and is concerned about myopathy. They have performed a CK test which is normal and recent fasting lipid profile reveals TC 4.5, LDL-C 2.2. There is no muscle weakness and the patient feels that the symptoms are currently tolerable.**

    What do you recommend?

    A. Stop simvastatin and substitute with ezetimibe
    B. Reduce simvastatin to 40 mg and assess progress
    C. Substitute simvastatin with atorvastatin
    D. Reduce simvastatin and add fibrate
    E. Encourage continuation of current treatment

15. **A 73-year-old woman has been given a fasting lipid test by her GP (TC 6.2, LDL 3.8). She feels that she has put on weight recently as a result of a general lack of energy and activity. The GP started simvastatin 40 mg nocte but the patient stopped it because she felt that it caused constipation.**

    What do you recommend?

    A. Investigate for secondary hypercholesterolaemia
    B. Lifestyle advice, 30 minutes exercise five times per week, and consider referral to dietician
    C. Encourage simvastatin re-initiation and advise that constipation is unlikely to be due to the statin
    D. Advise an alternative lipid-lowering drug such as ezetimibe
    E. Trial an alternative statin

16. **Which one of the following drug mechanisms of action is true?**

    A. Ezetimibe—cholesterol absorption inhibitor
    B. Simvastatin—bile acid sequestrant
    C. Cholestyramine—agonist of PPAR-α
    D. Nicotinic acid—intestinal cholesterol binder
    E. Gemfibrozil—HMG-CoA reductase inhibitor

17. A patient is not achieving target LDL-C on high-dose statin alone.

Which combination with statin is not recommended?

A. Gemfibrozil

B. Ezetimibe

C. Colesevelam

D. Nicotinic acid

E. Phytosterols

18. Which one of the following agents will have the greatest LDL-C-lowering effect?

A. Atorvastatin 40 mg od

B. Pravastatin 40 mg od

C. Simvastatin 40 mg od

D. Cholestyramine 8 mg od

E. Gemfibrozil 600 mg bd

19. A 20-year-old man is referred with tendon xanthomas and an LDL-C of 13 mmol/L.

What is the likely diagnosis?

A. Heterozygous familial hypercholesterolaemia (FH)

B. Homozygous FH

C. Familial combined hyperlipidaemia

D. Familial dysbetalipoproteinaemia

E. Familial lipoprotein lipase deficiency

20. A 33-year-old man attends clinic with a total cholesterol of 7.8 (LDL-C 5.1). He has no evidence of premature atherosclerosis or clinical xanthomata/xanthelasma. He volunteers that two uncles on the maternal side had heart attacks in their forties.

According to the Simon Broome criteria:

A. He has a definite diagnosis of FH

B. He has a possible diagnosis of FH

C. FH is ruled out

D. Fasting HDL-C and triglycerides should be measured for a diagnosis

E. Two further confirmatory lipid profiles are required

21. **A 17-year-old female presents with a 3-month history of progressive dyspnoea and fatigue. Her menstrual periods had become erratic. Examination revealed a loud first heart sound and multiple spotty pigmented areas around the face and shoulders. Full blood count, renal function, and thyroid function tests are normal. Her chest radiograph is unremarkable. A transthoracic echocardiogram is performed and shows a 4 × 5 cm smooth heterogenous pedunculated mass arising from the intra-atrial septum.**

    Which one of the following statements regarding atrial myxoma is true?

    A. Addison's disease is a common association with atrial myxoma

    B. Atrial myxomas rarely grow to >3 cm in diameter

    C. Atrial myxomas have a right to left ratio of 4:1

    D. Carney syndrome accounts for 7% of all cardiac myxomas

    E. The mass in the atrium is solid and avascular

22. **A 77-year-old female is seen 5 days after a right-sided ischaemic cerebrovascular event. There was a history of hypertension but no other significant cardiovascular risk factors. Examination revealed a resolving left hemiparesis and homonemous hemianopia. Cardiovascular examination was unremarkable. There were no peripheral stigmata of endocarditis. CRP was 17 and WCC 10.4. Urinalysis showed 1+ protein. Five days of cardiac monitoring showed sinus rhythm. A transthoracic echocardiogram is shown in Figure 10.3.**

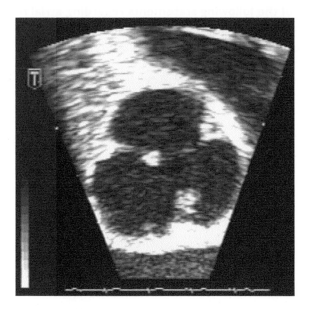

Figure 10.3

Which one of the following statements is correct?

A. There is no indication for blood cultures in this case

B. This tumour often presents with constitutional symptoms

C. Histologically, this tumour is similar to a Lambl excrescence

D. Surgery is not indicated unless there is haemodynamic compromise due to obstruction

E. These tumours are usually multiple and arise from the endomyocardium of the right ventricle

23. You are following up a 42-year-old female in outpatients who recently underwent surgical resection for a mass that was discovered during investigation of a large pericardial effusion. The histology report has confirmed the presence of a capillary haemangioma.

Which one of the following statements is correct?

A. Capillary haemangiomas are a capsulated tumour composed of small blood vessels resembling capillaries

B. Arteriovenous haemangioma is also known as a cirsoid aneurysm

C. CMR is of no value in differentiating histotype

D. There are four distinct histotypes of cardiac haemangioma

E. Females are four times more likely to be affected

24. You are asked to see a 67-year-old male who presents with chest pain and a chronic non-productive cough. The symptoms had been present for over 18 months and were not progressing. He denied any haemoptysis. He had no significant past medical history. Cardiovascular and respiratory examination was unremarkable. Routine blood tests were normal. A CT chest is shown in Figure 10.4.

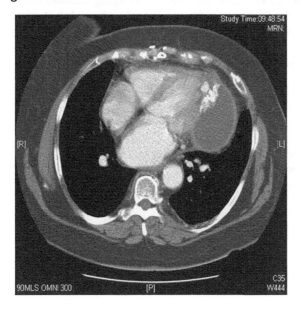

Figure 10.4

Which one of the following statements is correct?

A. Lung bullae can compress the right atrium

B. Percutaneous aspiration and ethanol sclerosis is a safe and effective treatment

C. Bronchoscopy is indicated

D. Calcification is a common finding

E. Cysts reach their maximum size by the early teens

25. **A 45-year-old male presents with syncope and progressive dyspnoea. He gives a 4-month history of progressive presyncopal episodes. A transthoracic echocardiogram and 24-hour Holter monitoring are performed. The Holter monitor demonstrates daytime periods of complete AV dissociation associated with his symptoms. The echocardiogram shows a 15 mm diameter mass arising from the inferior aspect of the right atrium.**

    Which one of the following statements is correct?

    A. The mean age of presentation of cystic tumours of the AV node is 60 years
    B. The cyst is located in the left atrium more frequently than in the right
    C. Cystic tumours are easily distinguishable from myxomas on echocardiography
    D. Cystic tumours of the AV node arise from endodermal remnants
    E. Cystic tumours of the AV node typically present with embolic phenomena

26. **You have been asked to see a 56-year-old male inpatient who presented 2 months previously with progressive shortness of breath and fever. He was discovered to have a large pericardial effusion which was tapped and was found to contain poorly differentiated cells. Subsequent CT imaging showed him to have widespread pulmonary metastasis with a 3 cm lobulated mass arising from and projecting into the right atrium, compressing the inferior vena cava. Biopsy tissue was obtained and confirms angiosarcoma.**

    Which one of the following statements is true?

    A. 2% of atrial myxoma can metastasize, typically to the lung
    B. The peak age of presentation is the sixth decade
    C. Angiosarcoma is typically symptomatic early in the disease process
    D. Angiosarcoma is most common in the left ventricle, arising from around the insertion of the posterior mitral valve
    E. Tumours showing mutations of the *TP53* gene have been described

27. **A 47-year-old female with known metastatic breast carcinoma has been admitted to the oncology ward for investigation of increasing shortness of breath. A pulmonary embolism was suspected on clinical grounds and a CT pulmonary angiogram was performed. It failed to demonstrate any pulmonary emboli but did show a 2.2 cm global pericardial effusion. On the basis of this, a transthoracic echocardiogram was performed which ruled out tamponade.**

    Which one of the following statements is correct?

    A. Breast carcinoma typically metastasizes to the pericardium but significant pericardial effusions are rare

    B. Lymphatic spread is more likely to metastasize to the myocardium, whereas haematological spread usually metastasizes to the pericardium

    C. Cardiac spread is unusual in malignant melanoma

    D. A constrictive picture can persist following pericardiocentesis

    E. Valvular metastases are a common finding in disseminated metastatic disease

28. **Regarding the prevalence of cardiac tumours:**

    A. The secondary to primary ratio is approximately 10:1

    B. Papillary fibroelastoma is the third most common of the primary benign cardiac tumours, behind myxoma and cardiac fibroma

    C. Lung carcimona is the most common metastatic cardiac tumour

    D. Although typically thought of as benign, 2% of atrial myxomas metastasize

    E. A male predominance of 1.4:1 is seen among the benign primary cardiac tumours

29. **A 57-year-old male patient is discovered to have an echogenic mass arising from the insertion point of the anterior mitral valve leaflet. He undergoes uneventful surgical resection. The mass is described as reddish and nodular. Frequent areas of calcification are identified by naked eye. Histologically, it is composed of oval CD34, CD31, and factor VIII positive cells consistent with epithelioid haemangioendothelioma.**

    Which one of the following five statements regarding this tumour is true?

    A. It is rare in females, with a male:female ratio of 20:1

    B. It is usually presented by the presence of metastases

    C. It typically occurs from the intra-atrial septum

    D. The differential diagnosis of adenocarcinoma is excluded by the presence of CD31, CD34, and factor VIII positive cells

    E. It often presents with complete heart block

1. A. Fabry disease is an X-linked condition. Therefore it will not be passed on from a father to his son (as he will receive the Y chromosome from his father).

2. B. The clinical scenario is typical of familial hypercholesterolaemia. Although *PCSK9* and *APOB* are causes, the most common cause is mutations in the low-density lipoprotein receptor. Sterol 27-hydroxylase causes cerebrotendinous xanthomatosis, and the low-density lipoprotein receptor adaptor protein 1 causes recessive hypercholesterolaemia.

3. C. He is affected with a dominantly inherited condition. Therefore there is 1 in 2 chance for each child.

4. A. The right ventricle is a common site for trabeculations occurring as a normal variant. All the other findings would raise concern that the trabeculations might represent pathological non-compaction.

5. A. Holt–Oram syndrome causes septal defects, AV node disease, and radial ray abnormalities, but not pulmonary stenosis. In addition, it is not associated with learning difficulties.

6. B. Although syncope is considered a risk factor, this is usually excluded when it occurred more than 10 years previously.

7. D. Widely spaced eyes (hypertelorism) is commonly seen in those with Loeys–Dietz syndrome but not with Marfan syndrome, familial aortic aneurysms, or other causes.

8. E. *KCNH2* is one of the more common causes of long QT syndrome and has not been associated with aortopathies.

9. E. *SCN5A*, the cardiac sodium channel, is associated with a broad range of conduction and arrhythmic disorders including long QT syndrome, Brugada syndrome, familial AF, and sick sinus syndrome. Catecholaminergic paroxysmal ventricular tachycardia is due to mutations in the cardiac ryanodine receptor, and recessively *CASQ*, which affect calcium release from the sarcoplasmic reticulum.

10. C. Hypertrophic cardiomyopathy is most commonly inherited in an autosomal dominant fashion due to sarcomere gene mutations. This is possible here; penetrance is incomplete, hence the unaffected female. X-linked inheritance with manifesting females is possible as there are no examples of male-to-male transmission; therefore Fabry disease is possible, although less likely. Transmission from a father to a child excludes a mitochondrial DNA mutation. Laminopathy is dominantly inherited but causes dilated cardiomyopathy with conduction defects.

11. D.   Diabetes is not part of the SCORE scoring system as these patients have already identified themselves as high risk and require intensive risk factor modification. Diabetic patients are defined as very high risk if there is evidence of end-organ damage or an additional CV risk factor.

12. D.   This diabetic patient already has evidence of end-organ damage reflected by microalbuminaemia. This identifies **very high** risk irrespective of other factors. Immediate drug therapy is indicated for LDL >1.8 (and should be considered even with very low LDL) with aggressive risk factor modification.

Other **very high** risk factors are chronic kidney disease (GFR < 30), established atherosclerotic disease (including carotid plaque), and a SCORE risk ≥10%.

The treatment target LDL-C is <1.8 (or at least 50% reduction) in these very high risk patients.

13. A.   Total cholesterol and LDL-C constitute the primary targets for treatment (as opposed to the protective HDL-C) primarily because of the large volume of compelling data and the fact that they can be modified with lifestyle changes and pharmacotherapy. The ESC recommends LDL-C targets which are graded to risk (<1.8 for very high risk, <2.5 for high risk, and <3.0 for moderate risk). JBS2 and NICE currently recommend TC <4.0 (LDL-C < 2.0). Therefore answer D can also be correct!

The ESC uses the SCORE chart to calculate CV death risk. Diabetes is not included in the risk charts and these individuals are assumed to be high risk (very high risk if evidence of end-organ damage). JBS2 charts calculate CV disease development risk, but JBS3 will include lifetime risk. JBS2 (2005) and NICE (2008) regard a 20% risk of developing CV disease over 10 years as high risk and the threshold for statin therapy for primary prevention.

14. C.   This patient is experiencing myalgia (occurs in 5–10% patients), but not myopathy, secondary to high-dose simvastatin. However, the patient has not achieved target cholesterol post MI. Atorvastatin is a more potent statin and may be better tolerated without requiring maximal titration. If the target is still not reached, combination therapy is appropriate.

15. A.   This patient has features of hypothyroidism which is associated with cholesterol elevation and is solved by thyroid correction. Secondary causes of hypercholesterolaemia should be considered prior to pharmacological intervention. These include:

- hypothyroidism
- nephrotic syndrome
- pregnancy
- Cushing's syndrome
- anorexia nervosa
- immunosuppressant agents
- corticosteriods.

16. A.   Ezetimibe inhibits intestinal uptake of dietary and biliary cholesterol without affecting the absorption of fat-soluble nutrients. Statins reduce synthesis of cholesterol in the liver by competitively inhibiting HMG-CoA reductase activity. The reduction in intracellular cholesterol concentration induces LDL receptor expression on the hepatocyte cell surface which results in extraction of LDL-C from the blood. Cholestyramine is a bile acid sequestrant. Gemfibrozil is a fibrate and an agonist of PPAR-α.

17. A.   Combination of statins with fibrates may enhance the risk for myopathy. The risk is highest with gemfibrozil, and the combination should be avoided. The risk appears to be small with other fibrates. Colesevelam is a newer bile acid sequestrant.

18. A.   Statins have the greatest effect on LDL-C followed by bile acid sequestrants and then fibrates (which have a greater effect on triglycerides): rosuvatatin > atorvastatin > simvastatin > pravastatin.

19. B.   The presence of tendon xanthomata is virtually diagnostic of FH. LDL-C concentrations >13mmol/L in adults is suggestive of a clinical diagnosis of homozygous FH, and DNA testing would be appropriate.

20. B.   Simon Broome criteria are used to make a diagnosis of FH in an index individual. In an adult, TC >7.5 (LDL-C >4.9) is suggestive of FH when associated with a family history of premature CV disease (or definitive family history of TC > 7.5). A definite diagnosis is made in the presence of tendon xanthoma (including in a family member) or DNA mutation (LDL-R, apo B-100, or *PCSK9*).

21. D.   Seven per cent of atrial myxomas occur as part of a complex called Carney syndrome. It typically comprises three features: myxoma (may be multiple) of the heart and skin, lentiginosis (hyperpigmentation of the skin), and endocrine overactivity (commonly Cushing's disease). It has been described under two different acronyms:

- NAME—naevi, atrial myxoma, myxoid neurofibroma, and ephelides
- LAMB—lentiginosis, atrial myxoma, mucocutaneous myxomas, and blue naevi.

The syndrome presents earlier than typical atrial myxoma and shows no female prevalence. The tumour tends to recur following surgery.

It is an autosomal dominantly inherited syndrome. A mutation in the putative tumour suppressor gene (*PRKAR1A*, 17q24) has been found.

22. C.   Papillary fibroelastomas are rare, representing <10% of all primary cardiac tumours. Ninety per cent occur on the valves, but they have been reported to arise on the intima of the right coronary sinus, the ventricles, and the mitral valve apparatus.

The majority (90%) are single, but multiple lesions have been described and are usually <1 cm in diameter. Left-sided fibroelastomas are more commonly reported than right-sided ones. Most patients are over 50 years of age. Clinical examination is typically unremarkable.

The potential for fibroelastomas to cause serious complications has been increasingly apparent. Fibroelastomas of the left side of the heart have been associated more frequently with serious symptoms. Cerebrovascular symptoms have been described frequently and many of these patients have had multiple episodes.

Some papillary fibroelastomas are congenital. However, most lesions are probably acquired. Some authors regard fibroelastomas as giant Lambl excrescences (Salyer WR), whereas others (McAllister and Fenoglio) regard them as true benign neoplasms.

The risk of embolic phenomenon is not well correlated with the size of the structure and for this reason it is generally thought that even small fibroelastomas should be considered for surgical resection.

23. A. Haemangiomas are benign and consist of an increased number of normal or abnormal blood vessels. They account for 5% of benign cardiac tumours and represent around 2% of all cardiac tumours. They are most frequent in young adults, and have an equal distribution between sexes.

Many are asymptomatic and are discovered as incidental findings during imaging. If significant intra-cavity projection occurs, haemangiomas are capable of causing obstructive symptoms. Haemangiomas can occur in any of the four cardiac chambers but have a predilection for the ventricles. Haemangiomas within the pericardium may present with pericarditis or pericardial effusions. Others present with constitutional symptoms; fever, weight loss, raised ESR and white cell count.

Histologically, haemangiomas can be broadly classified into three types.

1. Cavernous haemangiomas are composed of multiple dilated thin-walled vessels.

2. Capillary haemangiomas consist of very small vessels.

3. Arteriovenous haemangiomas are made up of dysplastic malformed arteries and veins.

Capillary haemangioma are capsulated whereas the other two types tend to be infiltrative.

CT is helpful in evaluating the extent of the tumour and invasion of adjacent structures whereas CMR is superior in histotype differentiation.

Treatment involves surgical resection of the lesion. For tumours involving important structures, incomplete resection may be inevitable. Resection allows a histological diagnosis, reduction of tumour mass, and improvement of clinical symptoms. Prognosis is generally very good and in most patients the tumours do not recur.

24. B. Congenital pericardial cysts are relatively frequent. They may be uni- or multilocular of diameter 1–15 cm and are full of serous fluid. Although most patients are asymptomatic, cysts may also present with chest pain, dyspnoea, palpitations, or cough. Although echocardiography is useful, additional imaging by CT or CMR is often needed. The treatment for symptomatic congenital cysts is percutaneous aspiration and ethanol sclerosis. If this is not feasible, video-assisted thoracotomy or surgical resection may be necessary.

Guidelines on the diagnosis and management of pericardial diseases: Executive Summary. Eur Heart J, 2004; 25: 587–610.

25. D. Cystic tumour of the atrioventricular node (also known as tawarioma) is very rare and classified as benign, although it may lead to significant morbidity and mortality due to obstruction, arrhythmias, and embolic phenomena. The mean age of clinical presentation is 40, and there is no sex predilection.

Cystic tumours usually consist of multicystic nodules and are located in the region of the AV node, in the triangle of Koch, on the right side of the intra-atrial septum in front of the coronary sinus.

Histologically the tumour is derived from endodermal remnants. It infiltrates and compresses the AV node leading to complete heart block (75%), incomplete heart block (15%), or sudden cardiac death (10%). The cysts, which are visible to the naked eye, are filled with a mucoid substance. This is a difficult tumour to identify on non-invasive studies or clinical findings. Treatment requires immediate surgery.

26. E. The most common of the primary cardiac malignant tumours, angiosarcoma is a tumour of endothelial cell differentiation. It is found in patients of all ages, with a peak in the fourth decade, and there is no sex predilection. The most common site is the right atrium. Angiosarcoma of the heart is considered primary if there is no evidence of previous or concomitant tumours in the soft tissue, bone, or subcutaneous tissue.

Presenting symptoms include fever, myalgia, and weight loss as well as chest pain and arrhythmias. In more advanced disease, lung metastasis, congestive heart failure, and large pericardial effusions can be seen.

Endomyocardial biopsy can provide in vivo diagnosis.

Echocardiography will demonstrate an irregular echogenic mass, typically associated with a pericardial effusion. Angiographically the mass can appear to be highly vascular. CT and CMR show the heterogeneity of the mass, including tissue necrosis and haemorrhage.

One-third of angiosarcomas are poorly differentiated, and two-thirds are moderately differentiated. Cells can express endothelial cell antigen (factor VIII, von Willebrand factor, CD31, and CD34), and mutations of the *TP53* and *K-ras* genes have been reported.

Mean survival is 10 months.

27. D. Cardiac metastases occur via four routes:

- lymphatic spread
- haematological spread
- direct infiltration
- transvenous extension.

Pericardial metastases typically arise from lymphatic spread whereas haematogenous spread preferentially gives rise to myocardial metastases. Endocardial tumour deposits are rarely found.

Owing to their location and prevalence, lung and breast carcinomas are the most common tumours causing cardiac metastases and both preferentially affect the pericardium, resulting in usually large effusions. Cardiac metastases are seen in around half the cases of metastatic melanoma.

Extracardiac tumours may reach the atria and ventricles by transvenous extension. Renal cell carcinoma growth through the inferior vena cava into the right atrium is thought to occur in up to 1% of cases. Rarely, bronchial carcinoma spreads through the pulmonary veins into the left-side heart cavities.

In cases of pericardial effusion causing circulatory embarrassment, pericardiocentesis is mandatory and may help diagnosis. Following pericardiocentesis, a constrictive picture often persists due to inflammation and thickening of the pericardium.

28. C. Cardiac tumours have a prevalence rate of 0.056% for primaries and 1.23% for secondaries, with an approximate ratio of secondary to primary of 20:1 (Lam KY).

The University of Padua has reported on an extensive post mortem series, which described 210 primary cardiac tumours, of which 89% were benign and 11% malignant. In this series, papillary fibroelastoma was the second most common benign primary cardiac tumour after atrial myxoma (Basso C).

Lung carcinoma is the most common metastatic cardiac tumour (approximately 33%). Lymphoma and leukaemia (16%) are the second most common followed by breast (5%), hepatic (5%), and kidney (4%) carcinomas.

Atrial myxoma is a benign disease that does not metastasize. It typically presents with constitutional, obstructive, or embolic symptoms.

In the primary benign cardiac tumours, there is a female predominance of 1.4:1. The mean age is 47 years.

29. D. Previously considered a low-grade or borderline malignant vascular lesion, epitheloid haemangioendothelioma is classified as a malignant tumour, along with angiosarcoma, because of its local aggressiveness and metastasizing potential. It is a very rare tumour.

There is a spectrum of disease with benign epithelioid haemangiomas at one end and the highly malignant epithelioid angiosarcoma at the other. The epithelioid haemangioendothelioma sits in the middle. Systemic metastasis is reported in approximately 20% of cases described in the medical literature (Lisy M). Treatment is radical surgical resection. There is limited value in radiotherapy and chemotherapy (Moulai N).

Originating from the subendocardium, these tumours can occur at any location within the heart. The expression of vascular endothelial markers, such as von Willebrand factor, CD31, and CD34, rules out metastatic adenocarcinoma or melanoma.

The prognosis is unpredictable and typically poor.

1. **You are looking after a 75-year-old man who was admitted 3 days previously with an anterior STEMI and underwent primary PCI to his LAD. He has made a good recovery and his echocardiogram shows that he has only mild LV impairment. He is asking about safe levels of physical activity once he goes home.**

   What should you advise him?

   A. To return immediately to his previous (pre-admission) level of activity
   B. That exercise is dangerous after a heart attack and he should continue with at least 2 weeks of bed rest after he returns home
   C. That he should be physically active for 20–30 minutes a day to the point of slight breathlessness
   D. That he should undertake a 30-minute warm up period prior to any exercise
   E. That he should start with at least 20–60 minutes of moderate aerobic exercise, three to five times a week

2. **One of your patients is about to be discharged following an NSTEMI. They ask you for some dietary advice to help to try and reduce their risk of having a further heart attack.**

   What advice should you give?

   A. To eat a Mediterranean-style diet with less meat and more bread, fruit, vegetables, and fish, and to replace butter and cheese with products based on vegetable and plant oils
   B. To read food labels when shopping to ensure that they reduce the amount of mono-unsaturated fats in their diet and eat more foods containing saturated fats
   C. To eat at least 1 g of omega-3 fatty acids, which are contained in oily fish, every week
   D. To take supplements containing beta-carotene, antioxidant supplements, (vitamin E and/or C), or folic acid to reduce cardiovascular risk
   E. All of the above

3. **You are reviewing a 60-year-old patient in clinic after a recent NSTEMI. They have not yet completed their cardiac rehabilitation programme and are asking for advice about ongoing physical activity. They have been looking online and have come across articles that say they should exercise at about 6 'METs'.**

    They ask you to explain what a MET is and if it means that they have to jog to keep healthy.

    A. 1 MET, or metabolic equivalent of task, is equivalent to the resting metabolic rate when sitting quietly, and has a conventional reference value of 3.5 mL O_2/kg/min which is equal to 1 kcal/kg/h

    B. 1 MET, or metabolic equivalent of task, is equivalent to the resting metabolic rate when sleeping, and has a conventional reference value of 3.5 ml O_2/kg/min which is equal to 1 kcal/kg/h

    C. 1 MET, or metabolic equivalent of task, is equivalent to the resting metabolic rate when sitting quietly, and has a conventional reference value of 6.5 mL O_2/kg/min which is equal to 1 kcal/kg/h

    D. 1 MET, or metabolic equivalent of task, is equivalent to the resting metabolic rate when sleeping, and has a conventional reference value of 6.5 mL O_2/kg/min which is equal to 1 kcal/kg/h

    E. The METs are a baseball team from New York that have sponsored an exercise programme for cardiac patients

4. **When advising patients about the DVLA regulations governing the entitlement to drive a private car or motorcycle, which one of the following statements is correct?**

    A. After an ACS successfully treated by PCI, patients can drive after 1 week providing that their ejection fraction is >15%

    B. After an elective PCI patients cannot drive for 24 hours

    C. After a CABG patients cannot drive for 4 weeks

    D. Patients with angina can continue driving even if symptoms occur at rest, with emotion, or at the wheel

    E. After an ACS for which treatment with PCI has been unsuccessful, patients can drive after 4 months

5. **Whilst you are working in your local cardiology ward, one of the nursing staff approaches you and asks, in general, which patients are very high risk and will need specialist assessment prior to referral for the exercise component of your local cardiac rehabilitation (CR) programme.**

    Which one of the following statements is correct?

    A. Patients with cyanotic congenital heart disease or those who have received an implantable cardiac defibrillator should never be referred for cardiac rehabilitation
    B. Patients with decompensated heart failure should be encouraged to exercise if it is part of a cardiac rehabilitation programme
    C. Patients with severe valvular stenoses can take part in exercise programmes whilst awaiting valve replacement surgery
    D. Patients who undergo exercise testing and develop angina at <5 METs are safe to participate in community-based exercise programmes
    E. Patients with angina or breathlessness occurring at a low level of exercise (e.g. inability to complete the first 4 minutes of the shuttle walking test) should participate in exercise sessions based in a safe environment with access to a defibrillator and staff trained in advanced life support

6. **You are working in a general cardiology clinic and are just finishing a consultation with a 69-year-old man who had been admitted with an NSTEMI 6 weeks previously. He has recovered well and has good LV function on a recent echocardiogram. His medications include aspirin, clopidogrel, bisoprolol, ramipril, and simvastatin. On the way out of the door he mentions some concerns about sexual dysfunction.**

    Which one of the following statements is incorrect?

    A. You are usually fit enough to have sex if you can comfortably walk about 300 yards on the flat, or climb two flights of stairs briskly without getting chest pain or becoming breathless
    B. Patients can resume sexual intercourse 4 weeks after an uncomplicated MI
    C. Erectile dysfunction is often due to underlying vascular disease, but can also relate to a patient's use of beta-blockers and/or ACE inhibitors
    D. Phosphodiesterase type 5 inhibitors (e.g. Viagra/sildenafil) could now be considered for use in this patient
    E. Patients on nitrates and/or nicorandil should avoid taking phosphodiesterase type 5 inhibitors because this can lead to dangerously low blood pressure

7. **When advising patients about the DVLA regulations governing the entitlement to drive a private car or motorcycle, which one of the following statements is incorrect?**
   A. After implantation of a standard permanent pacemaker patients may not drive for 1 week
   B. After implantation of a CRT-P device patients may not drive for 1 month
   C. After implantation of a prophylactic ICD patients may not drive for 1 month
   D. After the initial insertion of an ICD implanted for a ventricular arrhythmia associated with incapacity, patients may not drive for 6 months
   E. Patients with an ICD should stop driving for 1 month following any revision electrodes or alteration of anti-arrhythmic drug and for 1 week after a defibrillator box change

8. **When advising patients about the DVLA regulations governing Group 2 entitlement to drive an HGV, which one of the following statements is incorrect?**
   A. Patients with angina can be relicensed provided that they have been symptom free for more than 6 weeks, and can complete three stages/9 minutes of a Bruce protocol exercise tolerance test with no significant symptoms/ECG changes (having been off anti-anginals for 48 hours)
   B. After an acute MI, patients are disqualified from their Group 2 entitlement for 6 weeks. Thereafter they may be relicensed provided that they can complete three stages/9 minutes of a Bruce protocol exercise tolerance test with no significant symptoms/ECG changes (having been off anti-anginals for 48 hours)
   C. Following elective PCI, patients can resume their Group 2 entitlement after 1 week
   D. Following the implantation of a permanent pacemaker, patients are disqualified from their Group 2 entitlement for 6 weeks
   E. Following the implantation of an ICD, patients are permanently disqualified from their Group 2 entitlement

9. **You have been looking after an obese 55-year-old man with a history of hypertension, who was admitted with an NSTEMI.**

   Apart from optimizing his antihypertensive medication, which one of the following would be appropriate lifestyle advice measures for improving his blood pressure?
   A. Weight loss
   B. Reduction of his salt intake
   C. Regular exercise
   D. Stress management
   E. All of the above

10. **You are reviewing a 45-year-old man in clinic who suffered an NSTEMI 6 months previously. He has always led a healthy lifestyle, but when he was admitted he was found to have a cholesterol of 8.4 mmol/L. He is very concerned about his elevated cholesterol and is asking if there is anything he can do to help lower it.**

    You emphasize the importance of continuing with his statin medication, but which one of the following lifestyle measures would also be appropriate?

    A. Consuming saturated fats in preference to unsaturated fats
    B. Smoking cessation
    C. Reduce alcohol intake to 35 units per week
    D. Regular exercise with the aim of increasing waist circumference
    E. All of the above

11. **Your consultant has asked you to set up an audit of secondary prevention measures taken in your patients who have had an acute MI.**

    Which one of the following would be the correct standards/targets to assess?

    A. Eighty-five per cent of people discharged from hospital with a primary diagnosis of AMI or after coronary revascularization should be offered cardiac rehabilitation
    B. All patients should be offered treatment with aspirin, a statin, an ACE inhibitor/ARB, a beta-blocker, and an aldosterone antagonist post-MI unless contraindicated.
    C. A year after discharge, at least 80% of people should be non-smokers, exercise regularly, and have a BMI <35 kg/m^2
    D. Following a cardiac event, patients should aim for a target blood pressure of 150/90 mmHg
    E. Following a cardiac event, patients should aim to lower serum cholesterol concentrations to <5 mmol/L (LDL to <3 mmol/L)

12. **Cardiac rehabilitation programmes aim to consider the psychological and social implications of CHD as well as the practical lifestyle and medication measures involved in secondary prevention.**

    Which one of the following steps would not be an appropriate part of a cardiac rehabilitation programme?

    A. Assessment with the Hospital Anxiety and Depression Scale (HADS)
    B. Assessment of quality of life using the Dartmouth CO-OP Scales
    C. Assessment of quality of life using the Borg Scale
    D. Support for economic, welfare, and housing issues
    E. Support and advice for stress management

13. **A newly qualified physiotherapist has started working on the cardiology ward and is interested in the exercise component of cardiac rehabilitation.**

    Which one of the following statements would give correct information about the structured exercise component of the CR programme?

    A. Exercise sessions should involve low to moderate intensity activity at least five times a week for a minimum of 12 weeks
    B. Patients should be prescribed an individualized exercise regime
    C. Patients should not undertake resistance training
    D. Exercise sessions usually last 1 hour including an aerobic phase for 45 minutes and a period of relaxation
    E. Patients should be advised to aim for a perceived level of exertion of >15 on the Borg Scale

14. **The National Audit of Cardiac Rehabilitation has highlighted the problem of poor uptake of CR, with a mean of 41% of the target population taking part in 2008–2009.**

    Which one of the following statements is correct with regard to efforts to improve access to CR services?

    A. Sessions should be held in more accessible community venues or transport provided whenever possible
    B. Services should be able to adapt to an individual patient's gender, age, ethnicity, and mental and physical comorbidities
    C. Evidence shows that uptake is particularly poor amongst women, the elderly, people from ethnic minority groups, and patients from lower socioeconomic groups
    D. There is a need for improved referral from cardiology acute services
    E. All of the above

15. **You are asked to help develop CR services in your area with the resources available.**

    Which one of the following patient groups should be prioritized to receive support from the CR programme?

    A. Patients newly diagnosed with chronic heart failure
    B. Patients recently admitted with an ACS
    C. Heart failure patients who have had a step change in their clinical condition
    D. All patients undergoing reperfusion (e.g. CABG or stenting)
    E. All of the above

16. **You have been asked to help with the development and review of local CR services. As part of the programme the patients should receive a range of baseline measurements to help inform their goals and subsequently to assess them for change post-rehabilitation.**

    Which one of the following is not a baseline measurement recommended by the Department of Health?

    A. Psychological wellbeing (e.g. HADs)
    B. Echocardiogram
    C. BMI measurement or waist circumference
    D. Functional capacity (e.g. shuttle walking test, six-minute walking test)
    E. Quality of life (e.g. Dartmouth CO-OP Scale)

17. **You are working on a general cardiology ward, looking after a 55-year-old man who presented with an NSTEMI. The patient lectures on physiology at the local university and asks you about targets he should aim to achieve given his recent diagnosis.**

    Which one of the following would not be appropriate?

    A. Smoking cessation
    B. At least 20–60 minutes of moderate aerobic exercise three to five times a week
    C. A target blood pressure of 140/90 mmHg (or 130/80 mmHg in patients with diabetes or renal disease)
    D. A total cholesterol of <4 mmol/L and LDL cholesterol <2 mmol/L
    E. A 2000 calorie per day diet

18. **You are looking after a 75-year-old man who has been newly diagnosed with chronic heart failure.**

    As part of a referral to the CR services, which one of the following should not be considered?

    A. Fluid status (weight, postural BP) and management with diuretics
    B. Quality of life score
    C. Cardioprotective medication and device therapy (ICD, CRT)
    D. Functional capacity
    E. Psychosocial wellbeing

19. **You are working on a cardiology ward in a district general hospital and have been asked to teach the medical students about cardiac rehabilitation. A particularly keen student asks about the physiological mechanisms for the cardiac benefits of exercise.**

    Which one of the following statements is incorrect?

    A. On a microvascular level there is improved endothelium-dependent vasodilation, with decreased expression and activity of endothelial NO synthase

    B. Exercise causes changes in the autonomic nervous system which reduce the resting sympathicoadrenergic tone

    C. In patients with heart failure, as well as the benefits of exercise training already listed, studies have shown a reduction in circulating levels of angiotensin II, aldosterone, and atrial natriuretic peptide

    D. Exercise induces modifications within the renin–angiotensin–aldosterone system which result in reduced plasma renin activity

    E. Patients with chronic heart failure benefit from better respiratory function and improved skeletal muscle metabolism and function

20. **You are working on a cardiology ward in a district general hospital and have been asked to teach the medical students about cardiac rehabilitation. One of the students asks if there is an evidence base to support the role of CR.**

    Which one of the following is the correct response?

    A. The evidence is anecdotal but patients like it

    B. There is a moderate level of evidence with some randomized controlled trials suggesting efficacy

    C. There is good evidence for CR in patients with ACS, but the role of CR in chronic heart failure patients is based only on the extrapolation of this data

    D. There is a strong evidence base with many randomized controlled trials and meta-analyses supporting clinical and cost effectiveness

    E. There is better evidence for PCI in terms of life-years gained

CARDIAC REHABILITATION

1. C. Following an acute MI patients should be referred to the CR team for assessment, and in the meantime they are advised to be physically active for 20–30 minutes a day to the point of slight breathlessness. A warm-up period of 6–10 minutes should be encouraged as it allows the body to adjust to increasing demand. The main 20–30 minutes of activity should be at a moderate level of exertion and is best followed by a cool-down period which is often similar to the warm-up. Patients who are not achieving this should be advised to increase their activity in a gradual step-by-step way. After completion of their CR programme patients should be given long-term advice to continue with at least 20–60 minutes of moderate aerobic exercise three to five times a week.

2. A. Patients should be encouraged to eat a Mediterranean-style diet (more bread, fruit, vegetables, and fish; less meat; replace butter and cheese with products based on vegetable and plant oils). A healthy diet should include five portions of fruit and vegetables per day and patients should reduce the intake of salt and saturated fats. Post-MI patients should eat at least 7 g of omega-3 fatty acids per week (two to four portions of oily fish), and if they are not achieving this you should consider providing at least 1 g of omega-3-acid ethyl esters daily (as per the current NICE guidance, although this may be reviewed with the results of the Alpha Omega trial that shows a less clear benefit from omega-3 fatty acids). Patients should be advised not to take supplements containing beta-carotene, antioxidant supplements (vitamin E and/or C), or folic acid to reduce cardiovascular risk.

3. A. A metabolic equivalent is a way of expressing the metabolic energy requirements of a task as multiples of the resting metabolic rate (RMR). 1 MET is equivalent to the RMR when sitting quietly, and has a conventional reference value of 3.5 mL O_2/kg/min which is equal to 1 kcal/kg/h.

Jogging is equivalent to 7 METs and is not required to maintain fitness in this age group. Brisk walking with a lightweight pack or on hilly terrain is an appropriate activity, as is cycling on the flat.

4. C. Patients with angina should stop driving if symptoms occur at rest, with emotion, or at the wheel. Following an ACS, patients who have undergone successful PCI may drive after 1 week provided that no other urgent revascularization is planned and that their LVEF is >40% pre-discharge. Patients with an ACS who have not successfully been treated by PCI can drive after 4 weeks. Patients can drive 1 week after an elective PCI and 4 weeks after a CABG.

5. E. CR should be offered to all patients following an acute MI and those undergoing a CABG or angioplasty. CR should also be offered to patients with chronic heart failure and unstable angina with disabling symptoms. Increasingly there is also evidence to support the benefit for other patient groups including those with congenital heart disease, post cardiac transplantation, and those with implantable cardiac defibrillators. High-risk patients should participate in exercise sessions based in a safe environment with access to a defibrillator and staff trained in advanced life support.

High-risk patients include those with:

- a myocardial infarction complicated by heart failure, cardiogenic shock, and/or complex ventricular arrhythmias
- angina or breathlessness occurring at a low level of exercise (inability to complete the first 4 minutes of the shuttle walking test)
- ST segment depression ≥1 mm on resting ECG
- exercise testing with marked ST depression ≥2 mm or angina at <5 METs (3 minutes of a Bruce protocol).

Patients unsuitable for exercise training include those with:

- decompensated heart failure
- severe valvular stenosis or regurgitation
- refractory arrhythmias
- other clinical conditions which worsen with exertion.

6. D. Whilst the rest of the advice given in the options in the question is correct, phosphodiesterase type 5 inhibitors may be considered in stable patients who have had an MI more than 6 months earlier.

7. B. As with standard bradycardia pacemakers, patients who have received a CRT-P device should not drive for 1 week after implantation.

Patients with an ICD implanted for a ventricular arrhythmia associated with incapacity should not drive for 6 months after the first implant, for 6 months after any shock therapy and/or symptomatic anti-tachycardia pacing, and for 2 years after any therapy accompanied by incapacity. If the shocks were due to an inappropriate cause, patients can resume driving 1 month after these problems have been resolved. If the shocks were appropriate, and appropriate steps have been taken to prevent recurrence, patients can resume driving after 6 months.

Patients with an ICD implanted for a ventricular arrhythmia which did not cause incapacity can drive 1 month after ICD implantation, provided that their LVEF is >35%, no fast VT is induced on an electrophysiological study, and that any induced VT could be pace-terminated by the ICD twice, without acceleration, during the post-implantation study.

Patients with an ICD should stop driving for 1 month following any revision electrodes or alteration of anti-arrhythmic drug, and for 1 week after a defibrillator box change.

8. C. Patients who have undergone an elective PCI procedure are disqualified from their Group 2 entitlement for 6 weeks, and are required to meet the functional requirements in options A and B prior to relicensing. Following a CABG, patients are disqualified from their Group 2 entitlement for 3 months and may be considered for relicensing provided that their LVEF is >40% and the functional test requirements are met.

9. E. Following an MI, patients should aim for a target blood pressure of 140/90 mmHg (or 130/80 mmHg in patients with diabetes or renal disease). Lifestyle advice for hypertensive patients should include smoking cessation, weight loss and healthy diet regimes, reduction in salt intake, regular exercise, stress management, and keeping alcohol intake within recommended limits.

10. B. Following a cardiac event patients should aim for a total cholesterol of <4 mmol/L and LDL cholesterol <2 mmol/L (<1.8 mmol/L according to ESC) or a reduction of LDL-C by 30%, whichever is greater. In addition to continuing any prescribed medications, patients with elevated cholesterol can be advised to stop smoking, take regular exercise, keep alcohol intake within recommended limits (<21 units/week for men and <14 units/week for women), lose weight/reduce waist circumference, and maintain a diet low in saturated fat. It is important for diabetic patients to maintain their target HbA1c.

11. A. The National Service Framework for Coronary Heart Disease (NSF CHD) has set the target that 85% of people discharged from hospital with a primary diagnosis of acute MI or after coronary revascularization should be offered cardiac rehabilitation, and that 1 year after discharge at least 80% of people should be non-smokers, exercise regularly, and have a BMI <30 kg/m^2. NICE and ESC guidelines recommend that post-MI patients should aim for a target BP of <140/90 mmHg and a target cholesterol of <4 mmol/L (and LDL of <2 mmol/L (<1.8 mmol/L ESC)). All patients should be offered treatment with aspirin, a statin, an ACE inhibitor/ARB, and a beta-blocker. Patients should receive dual antiplatelets12 months following an ACS irrespective of angioplasty or the type of stent. Patients with signs or symptoms of heart failure and EF <40% (EPHESUS trial) should be offered treatment with an aldosterone antagonist.

12. C. The Borg Scale is used to assess the rate of perceived exertion, not quality of life. There are two Borg Scale systems—the original scale rates exertion from 6 to 20 compared with range 0–10 for the Borg CR10 Scale. The odd range of 6–20 is to follow the general heart rate of a healthy adult by multiplying by 10. The other measures listed in the question should be included in a CR programme, along with practical advice on return to work, driving, travel (including air travel), and return to sexual intercourse.

13. B. Exercise sessions should involve moderate-intensity aerobic activity at least twice a week for a minimum of 8 weeks. Resistance training is an integral part of rehabilitation exercise. Exercise sessions usually last for 1 hour including a 10–15-minute warm up, an aerobic phase for 20–30 minutes, and a 10-minute cool-down. Patients should be prescribed an individualized exercise regime.

Exercise intensity can be monitored using a pulse monitor or by manual pulse-taking, and looking at a percentage of the acquired maximal heart rate or estimated maximal age-predicated heart rate. Rating of perceived level of exertion is encouraged using the Borg Scale (either the 6–20 scale or the CR10 scale). When using the Borg Scale, low to moderate exertion corresponds to a score of 11–13 (4–6); a score of 15 (7) or more would indicate a high level of exertion.

14. E. The statements are all correct. Improving accessibility to rehabilitation services is vital. Greater referral (i.e. opt-out approach) is essential. Flexibility in provision is important, and patients should be offered the choice of hospital-, community-, or home-based programmes. Services should be culturally sensitive, with bilingual team members if required, and resources should be available for the visually and hearing impaired.

15. E. As a matter of priority CR should be offered to all patients who have had an acute coronary syndrome (including STEMI, NSTEMI, and unstable angina), those patients undergoing reperfusion via either CABG or PCI, and patients newly diagnosed with chronic heart failure or with a step change in the clinical presentation of their condition. Increasingly there is also evidence to support the benefit for other patient groups, including patients with stable angina, with congenital heart disease, following cardiac transplantation, and with implantable cardiac defibrillators or ventricular assist devices.

16. B. Although NICE guidelines for secondary prevention following myocardial infarction and chronic heart failure recommend the assessment of left cardiac function using echocardiography, this is not an assessment against which to assess change post-CR. These measures include:

- psychological wellbeing (HADS)
- functional capacity/fitness (shuttle walk test, six-minute walk test, etc)
- BMI measures for all patients
- quality of life (Dartmouth CO-OP or Minnesota Living with Heart Failure (MLWHF) tests)
- smoking cessation
- compliance with medication
- compliance with a healthy eating plan.

17. E. Following an ACS, patients should be counselled to set realistic individualized goals. However, recommended targets include:

- smoking cessation
- at least 20–60 minutes of moderate aerobic exercise three to five times a week
- target blood pressure of 140/90 mmHg (or 130/80 mmHg in patients with diabetes or renal disease)
- total cholesterol of <4 mmol/L and LDL cholesterol <2 mmol/L (even if premorbid cholesterol levels are low, patients will still benefit from reducing their cholesterol by 25% (LDL-C by 30%)).

The NSF CHD has set the goal that 1 year after discharge, at least 50% of people should be non-smokers, exercise regularly, and have a BMI <30 kg/m^2.

18. B. The core components of CR are the same for patients with chronic heart failure as for patients following an ACS. These include lifestyle measures (e.g. smoking, diet, and exercise/functional capacity), risk factor management (BP, lipid and blood sugar control), cardioprotective drugs and devices, and psychosocial wellbeing. These core components are underpinned by education and long-term management strategies. In patients with chronic heart failure, it is also particularly important to assess fluid status and manage this appropriately with diuretics.

19. A. There is increased expression of NO synthase.

Exercise training has several neurohormonal effects. Changes in the autonomic nervous system reduce the resting sympathicoadrenergic tone, and modifications within the renin–angiotensin–aldosterone system result in reduced plasma renin activity. On a microvascular level there is improved endothelium-dependent vasodilation, with increased expression and activity of endothelial NO synthase, as well as increased angiogenesis and collateralization.

In patients with heart failure, as well as the benefits of exercise training listed in the question, studies have shown a reduction in circulating levels of angiotensin II, aldosterone, and atrial natriuretic peptide. These patients also benefit from better respiratory function and improved skeletal muscle metabolism and function.

20. D. A Cochrane review of exercise training (Jolliffe et al. 2001, updated in 2009) demonstrated that exercise-only cardiac rehabilitation and comprehensive CR reduced all-cause mortality by 27% and 13%, respectively, and cardiac death by 31% and 26%, respectively, for patients with previous MI, revascularization, or angina. There was no effect on non-fatal MI alone and there was no apparent additional benefit from comprehensive CR. The population studied included predominantly younger low-risk male patients.

A Cochrane review of studies of exercised-based CR in patients with mild to moderate heart failure (Davies et al. 2010) demonstrated a 28% reduction in heart-failure-related hospital admissions and an improvement in patients' quality of life, although no significant reduction in all-cause mortality was shown.

Davies EJ, Moxham T, Rees K, et al. Exercise training for systolic heart failure: Cochrane systematic review and meta-analysis. Eur J Heart Failure 2010; 12: 706–15.

Jolliffe J, Rees K, Taylor RRS, Thompson DR, Oldridge N, Ebrahim S. Exercise-based rehabilitation for coronary heart disease. Cochrane Database Syst Rev, 2001; (1): CD001800.

INDEX